Finding Work
In Global Health

Finding Work
in Global Health

*A Practical Guide for Jobseekers—or Anyone Who
Wants to Make the World a Healthier Place*

Garth Osborn and Patricia Ohmans

Health Advocates Press
Saint Paul, Minnesota

Finding Work in Global Health
A Practical Guide for Jobseekers

Published by Health Advocates Press
a division of Health Advocates
843 Van Buren Avenue
Saint Paul, Minnesota 55104
651-489-4238

Second Paperback Edition 2005

Library of Congress Cataloging-in-Publication Data
Osborn, Garth 2005
        Finding Work in Global Health: A Practical Guide for Jobseekers
        or Anyone Who Wants to Make the World a Healthier Place/
        Garth Osborn and Patricia Ohmans
        2nd edition p.cm.

ISBN 0-96756061-6
1. International heath   2. Employment
I. Ohmans, Patricia II. Title

Book design by Patricia Ohmans; cover by Anthony Schmitz
Cover photos by Matt Bogenschultz

Printed and distributed in the United States of America
by BookMobile, Inc.
St Louis Park, Minnesota

This book is available at a special quantity discount for bulk purchase for sales promotions, non-profit fundraising, and educational purposes. Special books or excerpts can also be created to fit specific needs. For details, write Health Advocates Press Special Markets, 843 Van Buren Avenue, Saint Paul, MN 55104, or call 651-489-4238.

Thanks

The authors would like to thank the individuals profiled in this book, who kindly shared their insights and experiences.

Thanks are also due to Carol Berg, Debra Ehret, Arlen Erdahl, Bert Hirschhorn, Stacy King and Huy Pham for their careful reading and editorial suggestions.

Jeanne Freiburg, Nancy Miller, Lauren Panetta, Melanie Myers, Timothy O'Hearn, Joan Pasiuk, James Setzer, Robert Veninga, Bridget Votel and Reese Welsh offered important and useful information along the way. Don Leeper provided us with a crash course in publishing. Matt Bogenschultz kindly loaned us the cover photographs.

Finally, many thanks to Anthony Schmitz and to Lang Osborn, who provided invaluable support at every step.

To you

This book is dedicated to all those who carry out the good and necessary work of health care around the world.

From NILS DAULAIRE, MD, MPH
President and CEO, Global Health Council
"This is a terrific place to start"

It shouldn't be this hard, but finding work in global health for the first time is a bit like finding a coffee shop in Cairo without a map or translator. You know it's out there, but it's hard to figure out just where to start.

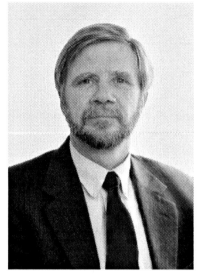

Global health is truly an eclectic field without any clearly defined career track. My first experience in the developing world happened almost by accident - while I was in medical school, a senior resident in pediatrics said he thought I might find working for an indigenous NGO that he knew in Bangladesh to be an interesting experience if I was willing to take a chance. I was, and have never looked back. Still, getting my first real job in global health after I had finished my training seemed like it would never happen. Ultimately it came about as a result of an evening spent playing hearts with some friends who happened to mention they had heard about a job in West Africa in what was gently described as "difficult circumstances." Again, I was willing to take a chance.

It seems most career opportunities I know in this field are a bit like that - random, almost chaotic. So how can anyone plan for that, make the most of what you have to offer, be prepared when the opportunity presents itself?

As the head of the Global Health Council, whose members include thousands of individuals and organizations on the front lines of global health, I get calls and emails on an almost daily basis from students, young professionals, and deeply caring individuals who want to know how they can help, and where they can begin to get some real-life experiences in the field. Unfortunately, career counseling is not what our members hired me for, and usually I can only refer them to groups who might offer field placements and wish them the best.

When I first read <u>Finding Work in Global Health,</u> I felt like I was reading the Lonely Planet guide to the life and career I have chosen. In approachable, human and humorous ways, Garth Osborn and Patricia Ohmans lay out the context, the scene, and some very practical advice that I wish I had had when I was first getting into this line of work. I enthusiastically concur that this is a terrific place to start for those looking to make a difference in global health. Who knows where it will take you? Just hang on for the ride of your life!

Contents

INTRODUCTION
The Right Work for You

So you want to go overseas and help people in need.

Perhaps you imagine yourself in a refugee camp, treating cholera victims. Or on horseback in the mountains, helping to immunize children. Perhaps you think you have some technical expertise that can help train government health workers. Or maybe you just know you want to help, somehow.

Whatever your global health dream is, congratulations! You are envisioning work for yourself that can bring meaning, challenge and excitement to your life and make a real difference in the lives of others.

But where should you begin to pursue your dream? And how can you find the right work to fit your life, your skills and your experience?

The right job for you

Fnding the perfect international health position is complicated. You can't just telephone one of the thousand US-based international health organizations and tell them you're ready to go.

The global health field is an increasingly complex one, with fierce competition for positions, many of which require specific skills, prior training and extensive experience. Every month, global health organizations receive thousands of unsolicited calls and letters from doctors, nurses, students and others wanting to work or volunteer overseas. Most posted positions get over 100 applications!

But don't despair. The perfect international health position is out there for you, whether you are interested in being a short-term volunteer, or you are trying to shape a life-long career. If you are willing to invest time and energy and follow the advice in this book, you can turn that investment into a lifetime of rewarding work.

How this book can help

Whether you've just begun to ponder going overseas or you've already begun researching the vast array of options open to you, this book will help you to:

- understand the field of international health: who's involved, what they're doing, and who's hiring;
- clarify your needs and what you expect to achieve from your experience;
- build your network, the key to finding your perfect job;
- get the most difficult job: your first one; and
- prepare for going overseas and for your return.

How to read this book

Finding Work in Global Health flows in a logical sequence, starting you off with an overview of the global health field in the first two chapters, and then concentrating on what you'll need to know and do to find your place in the arena. We'll take you all the way to the airport, leaving you at the departure gate. In the last chapter, the book picks you up when you're ready to return to the US.

Chapters are linked, and ideas developed in earlier chapters will pop up again later. Hence, we recommend that you at least skim this book from cover to cover once, before zeroing in on a specific area.

Between chapters we've included interviews with nine remarkable people, global health veterans all. Their memories and insights provide a valuable first-hand picture of the variety of experiences one can have in this field.

About the authors

Who are Garth Osborn and Patricia Ohmans, anyway? Well, we're friends, work partners, public health professionals, and people who are vitally interested in the health of others around the world. Both of us have advanced degrees in public health, with specialties in health care administration and health education, respectively.

In writing this book, we drew on our academic training and on our own experiences in global health. Between the two of us, we've spent the better part of four decades living and working outside of the United States: Patricia in Latin America, Garth primarily in East Africa, Asia and Central America.

Garth has worked as a volunteer, employee and consultant in several international health organizations. Patricia specializes in health communication, and has worked extensively with immigrants and refugees in Minnesota.

Global health work appeals to both of us for many of the same reasons that it probably appeals to you—for the chance to help others; for the travel and learning opportunities; for the friendships that develop over a lifetime; and the insights that occur in a flash. In writing this book, we've come to realize anew what a great field global health is, and to feel truly enthusiastic about encouraging others to enter it.

A note on terms

If you're new to global health, there's a glossary of acronyms in the back of this book that can help you, but there are a couple of usages that should be clarified up front.

For starters, there's the difference between "international" and "global." While the words are pretty much synonymous, (and we use them *almost* interchangeably in this book) there is a distinction to be made. Besides being three syllables shorter, "global" health makes a nod to the implacable globalization of every aspect of our lives. In doing so, it acknowledges how truly interconnected the health of people in every nation is, whether wealthy and developed or poor and developing. From the eradication of smallpox to the spread of HIV; from the proliferation of landmines to the sale of tobacco; from border to border, the health of people around the globe is inextricably linked.

Then there's "volunteer" and "employee." When we refer to a global health "volunteer," we're generally talking about someone who is paid at least a stipend for work they do overseas. This book does cover true volunteer opportunities—the programs where you pay for the privilege of going overseas and helping out in some way, like building latrines or teaching English. But we concentrate on programs and opportunities that will at least allow you to break even as you help, so you can spend more than a week or two donating your time and service.

Finally, a note about acronyms. You might as well get used to it: global health is awash in initials, with acronyms for everything from organizations to management systems to diseases. In some circles spouting acronyms instead of English is a way to demonstrate one's vast knowledge and experience. We've tried not to show off that way, but let's face it, there are only so many times you're going to want to read the words "United Nations High Commissioner for Refugees" (UNHCR). At the back of the book is a list of the most common global health acronyms. Most are used in the book. Learn them and you, too, can sound like you know what you're talking about!

LINNEA SMITH
"Someone needed a doctor"

In some ways it isn't at all surprising that I wound up where I did, yet if I had been asked ten years earlier—or even one year, or even one week, before my first trip here—I would hardly have predicted that I would soon be deciding to spend years in the Peruvian Amazon.

In 1990 I was a 40-year old graduate of the University of Wisconsin Medical School with specialty training in internal medicine. After completing my residency, I had joined a small group practice in a small town in west-central Wisconsin. For three years I had been practicing medicine there quite happily.

After medical school, I finally had enough money to take international vacations. I was a member of the Nature Conservancy, and when their magazine showed up with an ad for a trip to the Amazon. "Visit the rain forest! Ride in dugout canoes! See tarantulas and blue morpho butterflies!" It was too good to pass up. I requested a brochure, which outlined a week at the Explorama ecotourism centers, lodges founded by an archaeologist-geologist-anthropologist who was one of the first Peace Corps

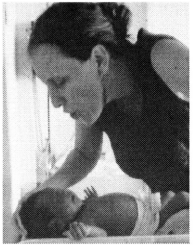

Linnea left her US medical practice to run a clinic on the Amazon River.

volunteers working at archaelogical sites in the Andes. It sounded good to me, so I signed up.

And an interesting trip it was. The week's vacation was filled with spectacular plants and animals: freshwater dolphins, anacondas, piranhas. We saw shooting stars and swam in the Amazon. One day we went for a long jungle walk. Lucio, our guide for the day, whose grandfather was a brujo —a shaman, or medicine man—pointed out many medicinal plants. There was one that he said is used for birth control. For this purpose, he explained, the sap is mixed with rum and sugar and left to ferment for three months. A woman drinks one shot glass of the concoction each morning before breakfast, for two weeks beginning just after her menses, and she becomes sterile, without any change in her menstrual periods. I wished I knew the physiology of that one. And we saw trees whose sap was reported to stop diarrhea, cure constipation, poison the intestinal parasites endemic to this place, and combat anemia—more amazing by the minute.

▲ ▲ ▲

After a week of incredible experiences, I had come to my last day on the Amazon. I was relaxing in my room when I heard someone shout, "She's in Room 40!" People were looking for me because someone needed a doctor. One of the lodge workers had been bitten by a fer-de-lance, a smaller, but still deadly relative of the bushmaster. The man had been cutting grass with a machete and had surprised the snake when he reached under the log where it was snoozing. The lodge possessed antivenin—two years past its expiration date, but probably still good— but someone was needed to administer it.

When I arrived, the patient looked calm but worried, with a piece of string tied loosely above his ankle. Despite the tourniquet, his foot was already red and swollen. While fifteen or twenty of the other employees and guides sat quietly around, lending support and contributing atmosphere, I popped the cap off the antivenin. It was a white powder in a small vial, requiring only sterile water to reconstitute it. I drew the water into the syringe, injected it into the vial and shook furiously (the vial, not me, personally!) Normally, one is supposed to administer a test dose of plain horse serum, because some people react violently, even fatally, to the antivenin. But since we had no test dose and since the patient was already numb up to the thigh, it seemed worth the risk to give the stuff.

Another shoestring was produced and tied above his elbow, while I upended the syringe and tapped out the air bubbles. Everyone was anxious and silent as I inserted the needle into his antecubital vein. The antivenin went in as I divided my attention between the slowly emptying syringe and the young man's face. Then I removed the makeshift tourniquet. There was no stethoscope, but by using a toilet paper tube as a crude substitute, I could hear a normal heartbeat and clear lungs. He was later taken by motorboat to the city, where he eventually recovered completely.

▲ ▲ ▲

I, however, did not recover. I already knew I wasn't ready for the trip to end. I awoke at dawn on the departure day, with the half moon directly above. I walked out and sat on the dock for the last morning of this vacation. I wasn't sure I wanted to go home. I found myself looking at that night sky filled with fireflies and lightning and thinking that if I had to leave this place, I would shrivel up and expire.

Once I reached home, it failed to feel any more like home. My instinct still said "Peru, Peru, Peru..." This feeling must seem rather strange to anyone who has not experienced it. You'd think that I would reflect on the decision, figure out various options, and make a thorough plan. After all, I didn't speak a word of Spanish beyond my three-word vocabulary. There was no support system for a physician there: no professional back-up, no laboratory or x-ray or pharmacy, not even a place in which to work. I had a wonderful practice in Wisconsin, not to mention a wonderful home where I had lived for nearly thirteen years. I told myself all of this, but none of it made any impression on my subconscious, which was now becoming conscious.

▲ ▲ ▲

I had given one of the lodge staff people my address and mentioned that I would be open to the idea of coming down to serve as the lodge doctor every now and then, should Explorama have such a need. Of course, I said, I couldn't leave my practice in Wisconsin but I thought I could get away for a few weeks or a month periodically. They took me up on the offer, and said they would provide me with one of the lodge's guest rooms *in which to offer medical services to local people, as well as to be on call for Explorama's guests.*

So it was that in May of 1990, armed with the contents of a doctor's black bag, one bottle of prenatal vitamins, a small microscope, and a three-month leave of absence from my Wisconsin practice, I returned to Peru. Certainly once I was here, I would come to my senses, find that the magic of the forest was not quite so compelling once I was actually living in it. Then I would go back to the life of a normal physician, in a normal practice, in a normal country.

Well, that's what I told myself.

▲ ▲ ▲

Editor's note: Of course, that's not what happened; instead, she stayed, and with the help of others, eventually built a full scale clinic near the lodge, where she still practices. For the full story of Linnea Smith's 15-year medical odyssey among the Yagua Indians of the Amazon Basin, be sure to read her memoir, *La Doctora: The Journal of an American Doctor Practicing Medicine on the Amazon River,* from which this selection is excerpted. *La Doctora* is distributed by the University of Minnesota Press; for more information, check her Amazon Medical Project website, www.amazonmedical.org.

CHAPTER ONE

The Top Ten Global Health Myths

Throughout its history, the field of international health has repeatedly redefined itself. These days, as we noted, even the name is changing, from "international health" to the zippier "global health." The days when a jungle doctor like Linnea Smith was the typical international health worker are fading fast. Global health practitioners today see as much heart disease and cancer as they do leprosy or snake bite.

Many other popular perceptions about global health work are also outdated or entirely inaccurate. Dispelling the myths below is your first step to understanding the field today.

Myth #1. The demand for global health professionals outweighs the supply.

The sad reality is that even though there is almost an infinite need for improved health care throughout the developing world, there are not enough paid positions for everyone who wants to work overseas. Paying your own way doesn't even guarantee you a position in international health, because the costs over and above your travel, room and board can be significant to the organization sending you.

Competition is also rife in academic training programs for those who want to study international health. Many university level international health programs receive three or four applications for every opening.

This is not to say that you can't find the perfect job or volunteer assignment, only that it's going to take thoughtful planning and persistence. The tips throughout this book, but especially in Chapter Six, "Landing that First Assignment," will help you search.

Myth #2. Working in global health is a good way to find yourself.

No! Drop this book immediately and proceed to the self help section of your local bookstore or library. Even a short assignment in global health is not the place to get over a bad marriage or to escape a floundering career. The physical and mental demands of living and working in a different culture can be daunting, even for those who have their act together. The purpose of international health should be to serve. Personal growth is inevitable, but it should not be your main motivation. (More on this later.)

Myth #3. You'll be able to treat patients.

Global health is moving away from sending doctors and nurses overseas to care for patients directly. Now more organizations are sending professionals overseas to provide training to strengthen local health care systems. Even orga-

TEN TOP GLOBAL HEALTH MYTHS

1. The demand for global health professionals outweighs the supply.
2. Working in global health is a good way to find yourself.
3. You'll be able to treat patients.
4. You must be a doctor or a nurse to work in global health.
5. Volunteering overseas will expand your technical skills.
6. As a health professional, the best way you can help those living in poor countries is to go there and offer your services.
7. Only developing countries suffer from underdevelopment in health care.
8. Most people in developing countries want and need modern western health care.
9. Knowing the answers means you can solve the problems.
10. More health care is the best solution to health problems in the developing world.

nizations that specialize in plastic surgery—typically short-term missions in which visiting surgeons try to operate on as many patients as possible—now incorporate training, for local surgeons to learn the latest techniques.

Myth #4. You must be a doctor or a nurse to work in global health.

A medical or nursing degree is a plus if you're interested in international health. But such training is only one route to being an effective global health professional. For example, the most common causes of child death in the developing world are dehydration, undernutrition, and infectious diseases. All are preventable or treatable without high tech equipment or extensive training.

It used to be that the "jungle doctor"—Albert Schweitzer,

Tom Dooley— was the epitome of the international health professional. But the focus has changed, from providing clinical services to training local people in low-cost, low-tech, high-impact skills which they can use in their communities. Skills like how to prepare and provide rehydration solution so children can survive bouts of diarrhea. Making sure women and children are immunized against the most common infectious diseases (such as pertussis, measles, tetanus, and diphtheria). Knowing where and how to dig wells and find potable water.

If you can demonstrate organizational and training skills, along with the ability to work in a cross-cultural environment, you've got assets that are just as valuable as medical school training. Read Chapter Five for more on the skills and experience employers are looking for.

Myth #5. Volunteering overseas will expand your technical skills.

In a word—yes and no. Yes, the experience of working in a developing country can affect the way you provide care for the rest of your career, even if you never set foot outside the US again. Witnessing the root causes of disease outside your own country can be the eye-opener of a lifetime.

But no, a community in a developing country is not a training ground to perfect your technical skills before going back to the US to work on "real" patients. Health workers who leave after a stint overseas and don't maintain connections can be viewed as opportunists by those who stay behind. Chapter Eight, on dealing with re-entry, suggests a number of ways to sustain important links and keep the lessons alive.

Myth #6. *As a health professional, the best way you can help those living in poor countries is to go there and offer your services.*
Maybe, but not necessarily. Not everybody can or should go overseas to work. This book will help you come to that decision. But if the decision is no, don't overlook what you can and should do from here to make life better for people in developing countries.

There are many positive things you can do, from donating money and expertise to an international humanitarian organization to lobbying our government for more international relief funding, or supporting corporations with ethical international trade practices.

Join the effort to ban land mines, lobby to stop the export of tobacco, or work to cease the unscrupulous promotion of infant formula in countries with unsafe water supplies. See Chapter Four for more on how to be a global citizen without leaving home.

Myth #7. *Only developing countries suffer from underdevelopment in health care.*
The days when you had to get on a plane or ship and go half way around the world to practice international health have passed. You can have a rewarding and effective global health experience right here in the US, probably in your own community, working to address many of the same challenges you would confront in a developing country.

Despite our enormous resources, the disparity in personal income in the US between the "haves" and the "have-nots" is greater than in any other industrialized nation in the world. Hundreds of thousands of people in the US are homeless. One in every five children lives at or below the poverty line. The US infant mortality rate, an important indicator for overall health within a society, falls behind many poorer countries such as Portugal or Korea. In addition, our inner cities and rural communities are facing increases in infectious disease and malnutrition, the leading causes of death in developing country children.

Want to work in global health without leaving the US? Try working with immigrant and refugee communities. Close to one million people come to the US every year, bringing with them their own health care beliefs and practices. The field of cross-cultural health has grown in response to the need for more culturally appropriate care and is increasingly recognized as an important component in the training of health professionals.

In fact, with the increase in cultural diversity in the US, there is a good argument for requiring all health science students to have an experience in global health or at least in a cross-cultural setting, as part of their training. Many international health practitioners who work intermittently overseas have chosen to focus their State-side work with immigrants and refugees. Check Chapter Four for more on how to think globally, but act locally.

Myth #8. Most people in developing countries want and need modern western health care.

The absence of a clinic or even a trained doctor or nurse in a village doesn't signal an absence of health care. Every culture on the planet has its own traditions for preventing illness and healing the sick and injured. Chances are good that these local beliefs have been practiced long before you will arrive in-country and will continue, long after you leave.

Promoting western style health care as the only alternative to local beliefs and practices can be the surest way of killing a project before it gets started. Many of the most effective global health projects have blended approaches and beliefs, rather than trying to replace them.

Myth #9. Knowing the answers means you can solve the problems.

Americans like to see challenges as problems to be solved. The room is dark; invent the light bulb. The mail is slow, invent the phone. The kids are bored; invent the TV (oops!).

This approach hasn't always worked well in the field of global health. There is probably a special place in heaven (or hell) for people whose clever international health projects didn't quite work out as planned. Solar powered ovens that didn't cook the food the way people were used to eating it. Water purification kits that left the water tasting funny. One classic case of good intentions gone awry was an immunization campaign poster that showed three simple panels, from left to right: a sick child, a vaccination syringe, and a well child. A great idea, right? Not in any country where people read from right to left!

Sometimes a community's health problems have simple solutions, or solutions that are more evident to an outsider. Often, they don't, for cultural reasons as well as technical ones. If a project doesn't fit within a community's culture, it may be doomed to fail.

Myth #10. More health care is the best solution to health problems in the developing world.

Much of the science we need to prevent and treat the leading causes of disease in the developing world is already

known to us. We can cure malnutrition, respiratory disease, malaria and tuberculosis, usually with cheap, simple
measures. The big challenge is how to expand access to all
those in need.

The solutions to world health inequalities often require
going beyond traditional curative health care to political
reform, human rights advocacy, economic development,
gender equity, and other arenas. Without fundamental
change in these areas, more health care will only mask the
real causes of illness.

CHERYL ROBERTSON
"You have to go to some tough places"

I grew up in California suburbs, a real suburban gal. I always wanted to see the world and be a part of it, but I grew up in a family that didn't do that. My mother's reaction when I invited her to come and visit me in Uganda (the first place I worked overseas) was "I'd rather be flogged!" My parents didn't discourage my travel interests, it just wasn't something that people like us did. But I was always interested in how other people lived. I majored in anthropology and got a nursing degree, but I knew I wanted to go overseas. I didn't really care where.

My first experience with going overseas was terrible. I was taking a class in international health, and a woman from an organzation called Minnesota International Health Volunteers showed up to guest lecture. At the end of her lecture she said "We're always looking for volunteers" and I raised my hand and said "sign me up." I'd applied for the Peace Corps but been turned down due to some past health problems. I knew very little about what I was getting into. It was really Gidget Goes to Uganda time.

▲ ▲ ▲

I arrived in Uganda in 1985 to find that it was in the midst of a low grade civil war. There I was, working in a small clinic just outside Kampala, the capital. It felt like I was working as a MASH nurse, taking care of wounded people, when I had signed on to do community health care. One afternoon I walked out behind the clinic and practically fell into an entire ditch filled with the skulls and bones of massacre victims. It was utterly horrifying.

A few weeks later, some co-workers and I went downtown one afternoon. We found after we finished our shopping that army tanks had rolled into town and were shooting the place up. A coup was going on. We literally hid behind a pile of wood on the sidewalk. We could see the Land Rover parked up the street, and watched the tanks finally drive by it, making an arc to get around it. We ran to the car and headed out of town. People were clinging to the sides, begging for a ride out of town. I had no idea what would happen next, but some of my Ugandan co-workers were pretty blase. One of them said, "As coups go, this one's awfully dull."

After a week, the American Embassy sent a car out to get us. They had organized an exodus and we had a half hour to get our stuff ready to go. Believe me, we were already packed, but we had terribly mixed feelings about leaving Ugandan colleagues behind. It was not just or ethical. We drove back into town—this after a week of bombing. You would not believe the devastation. You can see pictures, but it's nothing like the real thing.

It wasn't safe to leave the city, so we had to spend the night in a USAID safe house. That was even more surreal. This was a gorgeous house with gardens and greenery. The AID official served up some white wine and was listening to music: I remember the song, "We Are the World." We went out on the balcony that overlooked an overgrown golf course, and there were soldiers racing around shooting at one another on the green!

The next day we tried to drive out of Uganda. At the border, the soldiers at the checkpoint motioned all my friends out of the car and then made me stay. "No problem madam, you will be with your friends in 15 minutes," they said. Fifteen minutes came and went, and then an hour, and finally a whole day later I was still sitting in that car chainsmoking. Finally they let me go. That was my first international health experience!

▲ ▲ ▲

I couldn't let that be my memory though, so six months later, when Museveni overthrew the government, I asked to go back. This time I had the experience I was supposed to have. USAID child survival money flowed to the project I was working on, and suddenly instead of $10,000 we had $300,000 to spend. We had to get serious, really keep track and try to evaluate things.

When I returned, though, I began to see what kind of impact continual,

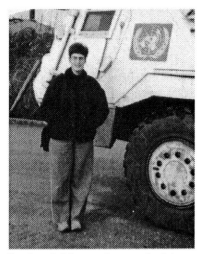

Cheryl studied how mothers sustain their families through war and trauma.

low-grade war has on people. It was hard for people to regain trust. The government talked about rebuilding the country, but many people were so traumatized that all they could do was hunker down and take care of themselves. In the area around Kasangati Clinic and in the Luweero Triangle, where I worked, more than 100,000 people had been killed. No one knew for sure how many. A huge number were also detained and tortured. People had been living in the bush, coming back to their homes at night to sleep if they could. It looks so familiar now seeing the news about Kosovo. I've learned that people do war the same all over.

And that realization probably led me to work at the Minnesota Center for Victims of Torture, which of course is all about regaining that trust for people. I went to Sarajevo during the Bosnian conflict to work with health professionals who were trying to set up similar rehabilitation centers for people who had been traumatized by torture.

▲ ▲ ▲

My husband and I adopted a son in 1988, and another son was born less than a year later, so for a while I was out of the international health business. I didn't go anywhere til 1992, when I made a conscious decision to make international health a part of my life again. My husband didn't really accept this for a while, and my younger son thinks the places I go are "icky," but my oldest is fascinated. I'm working on my PhD at the University now, exploring how women manage to mother in times of terrible stress like war, or in refugee camps. I've spent a lot of time in Bosnia.

Of course, when I went to Sarajevo in 1994 there was a war going on. I had to fly in on a UN transport plane, and ride into town in an armored vehicle. "Drop me off at the Holiday Inn," I said. This was where the embassies were and where all the foreign journalists lived, but it was completely dysfunctional. Half of the building was bombed away. Again I was very, very frightened, but I thought this was where all the people we'd trained through the Center for Victims of Torture had to be. The least I could do was to go to see them.

▲ ▲ ▲

I had some health problems when I was a kid and I was very protective of myself until I went to high school. As an adolescent, I was very worried about life and death stuff, more than normal. So it's funny that I do this work that people think of as high-risk. I don't think of myself as particularly adventurous and if I am, I'm a most fearful adventurer. But I am driven by a high level of curiosity about people outside my community. "How other people do it" has never stopped intriguing me. How do people make it through tough situations? To see that, you have to go to some tough places.

Editor's note: Since Cheryl was interviewed for the first edition of this book, she has completed her doctorate. She is now on the faculty in the School of Nursing at the University of Minnesota and continues her work with torture and trauma survivors.

CHAPTER TWO

What Is Global Health, Really?

If you've read Chapter One, you know that many of the perceptions people have of international health don't always correspond with reality. Understanding what global health really *is* will be crucial to finding a niche for yourself in this rapidly changing field.

In this chapter, we'll take a look at the current reality. We will:
- take you on a tour of headlines in global health history;
- introduce you to the major players in the field;
- provide some key definitions; and
- introduce six global health program models.

Be forewarned, this chapter is probably the densest one in the book. You may find it tough sledding, but persevere! By the end of the chapter, you should be ready to define your own place in the 21st century world of global health.

That was global health, then...

The current global health landscape (as seen from the US) developed through many of the shattering upheavals of the 20th century, but its origins go back to the mid-1800s. At the turn of the century, international health issues lay just beneath the surface of many of the major news stories of the day. Of course, the same is true today.

Picture these newspaper headlines:

In 1870:
Waves of Immigrant Laborers Bring Threat of Disease

From 1850 to 1950, the primary role of doctors and nurses was to treat Americans suffering from infectious disease. Throughout the early part of the century, fears that the growing number of immigrants arriving in the United States to work in factories, farms and mines were also carriers of tuberculosis, cholera and other contagious killers prompted medical researchers to look beyond national borders to prevent disease.

In 1907:
U.S. Growth and Trade Prospects Thwarted By Mosquito

As a growing empire, the US had a vested interest in curbing diseases that threatened its colonization of tropical countries. In the early 1900s, workers building the new Panama Canal sickened and died by the hundreds from mosquito-borne yellow fever. Working in Cuba, Dr. Walter Reed, a hero in infectious disease history for his discovery of the yellow fever vaccine, also helped build American awareness of the need to control "tropical" diseases.

In 1946:
Relief Efforts Concentrate On War-Torn European Cities

At the end of World War II, European cities were awash in survivors who desperately needed food, shelter and medical care, not to mention some hope that they might be united with their families someday. Major refugee assistance organizations such as the International Red Cross and the International Rescue Committee grew in response to the needs of these people. Their efforts continue today, sometimes even in the same Balkan countries ripped apart and reconstituted 60 years ago.

This is global health, now

In 1850, the world looked and felt like a loose collection of disconnected peoples. Over the intervening century and a half, expanded international communication, travel, commerce, and civilian-targeted conflict have torn down the barriers that kept communities in relative isolation.

First radio, then television, and now the internet have expanded access to information, even to those who live in closed societies. The ease of international travel has allowed more people to go from country to country with fewer restrictions. Free trade zones and global advertising have expanded markets, bringing consumer goods to every corner of the world where a profit can be turned. War has "evolved" from contained warfare between combatants to civilian-targeted conflict, leading to the traumatization of entire peoples as they flee across borders in search of safe haven.

These developments have changed the complexion of almost every country on the globe. The impact of these trends on health care has been revolutionary. Take a look at some of today's headlines:

AIDS, Tuberculosis and Other Infections Skyrocket:
Upsurge of Global Travel Blamed

Public Health Authorities Prepare Antidotes
for Biological Warfare Agents

Number of Refugees Fleeing Civil Strife
Worldwide Nears 20 Million

Internet and Television Give
Third World People "First World" Aspirations

We are bombarded daily with headlines like these and many others. At the turn of the millennium, the truly global nature of disease and health is undeniable.

But in fact, the *reality* of global health is different even from these headlines. Only the timely and dramatic seem to seep into the public consciousness, and then, only briefly. Here's a headline you probably *won't* see:

People Are Starving All Over the World

The fact that over 30,000 children die *every single day* from starvation and preventable illnesses is not news. There is enough food to feed every person on the planet. Most of the world's killer diseases are readily preventable and/or treatable. That's what should be news—but isn't. But then again, that's the *real* reality of global health.

Where the heck is Alma Ata?

We've explored what the public perception of international health is, and we've looked at the ways in which global realities shape and counter that perception. But how do global health practitioners themselves define what they're working toward? What mission—at least theoretically—do international health workers share?

The most widely accepted definition of the mission of international health comes from the 1979 International Conference on Primary Health Care at Alma Ata, in the former Soviet Union. This groundbreaking conference of world governments committed participant nations to achieving "Health for All by the Year 2000." Health was defined by the Conference in their *Declaration of Alma Ata* as "a state of complete physical, mental, and social well-being, and not merely the absence of disease or infirmity." (See the back of the book for the complete text; it's well worth reading.)

The Conference participants, a wonderfully idealistic lot, expressed the belief that health is "...a fundamental human right." The attainment of the highest possible level of health for every individual is "a most important worldwide goal whose realization requires the action of many other social and economic sectors in addition to the health sector."

Like the Bill of Rights or the United Nations Charter, the *Declaration of Alma Ata* sets a gold standard for achievement. Few nations have met the ambitious goals set forth in it, such as the eradication of malaria, or literacy levels for women that are equal to men. But the declaration's goals provide a workplan of sorts, and a yardstick against which progress toward global health can be measured. You might not hear many international relief workers quoting the Declaration of Alma Ata over beers at the local *cantina*, but rest assured that all but the most cynical of us have its noble goals in mind.

Global health players

When you think of someone involved in international health, who comes to mind? Albert Schweitzer in his Belgian Congo hospital? Mother Teresa ministering to the dying Untouchables of Calcutta? Chances are, you didn't name industrialist Henry Ford (whose Ford Foundation bankrolls thousands of health and development projects), or Carol Bellamy, Executive Director of UNICEF. And what about the millions of people in farms, villages and cities who are the recipients of global health and development efforts?

Individuals become involved in international health for a variety of reasons. These reasons are the stake that each individual (or group) holds in the success of a given international health initiative. Although health care providers are the direct *agents* of global health, they could never do their work without the involvement of at least three other sets of stakeholders: *donors, local governments,* and the recipient *communities* themselves.

For development to work, each stakeholder group has its own constituencies, needs and mandates which must be accommodated. This isn't just an abstraction; whatever your international health agenda is, you won't get far unless you are aware that others' agendas may differ substantially.

Say you've been hired by a US-based group to help set up a women's health program in a developing country, somewhere in Africa. Who will you need to accommodate and collaborate with in your efforts?

Donors: The money talks

First of all, you'll need to be aware of where your support comes from—and to be clear on who those *donors* are. Before embarking on any global health project (or accepting a job with a global health organization!) it's very wise to learn how the money talks, and what it says you should do.

The money to support global health work comes from a vast mix of sources, including United Nations-related agencies (also referred to as multilaterals), governments, private foundations, corporations, religious institutions, service organizations and individuals.

Each donor agency is driven by its own set of motivations that frame decisions on where to direct its support. Governments are often driven by national security concerns, guilt from colonial excesses, and interest in expanding trade opportunities and political influence. Corporations are concerned about their public relations image, expanding their market share, and access to a healthy work force. Motives of private funders range from religious zeal to political activism to personal interests.

Whatever the motivation, the donors' decisions have a profound impact on international health today, including the types of programs that get implemented, their location, the people served, and the organizations chosen to do the work.

Local governments: Overseers and implementers

To work effectively in a country, you must also understand the workings of the *local governing institutions.* It helps to have a big picture, even if you'll be working at the village level.

Local governments within developing countries have an important dual role in global health, as both overseers of the international organizations and program implementers. In the overseer role, they approve and coordinate the programs of the international organizations working within their geographic and administrative bailiwick, to make sure they are working in tandem with government rules and societal norms.

However, few developing country governments have the resources necessary to effectively oversee and coordinate these programs. In a few countries, nearly all the responsibility for the health sector has been delegated to international organizations. As a program implementer, developing country governments have competed with international organizations for funding so they can run the programs themselves.

Local communities: No longer passive

Finally, you must be familiar with the *communities* in which you will work. Traditionally, nothing more was expected of a community receiving international aid than to passively (but graciously) accept whatever assistance came from the outside. In reality, this never quite happened. Hundreds of failed development projects throughout the world are testimony to the fundamental role that a community must have in its own development.

Increasingly, community members themselves are becoming involved in the design, implementation and even the financing of the programs they receive. Community members are expected to sit on planning committees, donate their time as community health volunteers, and help find ways to meet the costs of sustaining health care services.

Program organizations: Where you come in

You may have noticed that we left out one group of people who hold an obvious stake in the success or failure of global health programs: the *program organizations* themselves. As you know by now, there are thousands of PVOs (private voluntary organizations); NGOs (local non-governmental organizations); local government agencies and academic programs that do much of the actual, day-to-day work of global health. They often compete fiercely for the support of donors and the approval of host country governments to implement their plans in developing countries.

The number of such organizations has exploded over the past 50 years, with over 1,000 international health organizations based in the US alone. Many developing countries host several hundred such international organizations, some of which have program budgets that dwarf those of the host country government.

Six ways to "do global health"

So what, exactly, is the work of global health? What do global health organizations and practitioners *do?* Several program "models" have grown out of the experience of the last 100 years. Below, we describe six of the most common ones.

Of course, borders between these various approaches have blurred as organizations incorporate the strongest components of each into their own programs. But read these descriptions with an eye to what *you* want to do.

1. Working with communities: primary health care

The Primary Health Care (PHC) movement grew out of the "Barefoot Doctors" who were a fundamental component of China's Cultural Revolution in the mid-1960s. It was based on the premise that the major causes of infant and child deaths and sickness (undernutrition, diarrheal diseases, pneumonia, and vaccine-preventable illnesses) in the developing world could be prevented or treated with simple, low cost measures that didn't require trained doctors or nurses. Health workers with only minimal training could bring these life-saving services to communities that had never seen a doctor or nurse.

The *Declaration of Alma Ata* of 1978 adopted community-based PHC as the approach to achieving its goal of "Health for All by the Year 2000." PHC programs have since been implemented throughout the world, in urban and rural communities as well as developing and industrialized countries.

PHC programs work with comunities, volunteers, NGOs and healthcare providers to prevent and treat the most common (and often the most dangerous) health problems. At their best, they are characterized by partnerships, collaboration, training, capacity building and health education. These programs can lead to expanded immunization coverage, the control of infectious disease, and increased access to family planning.

As a provider of PHC programs, you can help improve the health status of a community, through better family planning, immunizations, and treatment of diarrheal diseases with oral rehydration. But you will face major challenges with this program approach. These include covering the cost of supporting the community health workers; evaluating the success of the programs through solid data collection and analysis; and linking the lay health workers into the country's health care system, to make the project last.

2. Setting up safe havens: refugee relief

The United Nations defines a refugee as anyone "forced to flee their country based on a well-founded fear of persecution." Although they aren't part of the official count, there are also millions more people displaced from their homes by war or disaster, who are unable to leave their country. In refugee camps, international organizations and multilateral agencies (primarily the United Nations High Commissioner for Refugees, or UNHCR) provide the basic necessities, including food, health care and housing.

Health care programs are usually a mix of clinic or hospital-based care and community-based PHC programs. With the increase in international peace-keeping missions and multinational fighting forces since the late 1980s, the military has also become more involved in refugee situations, providing protection, infrastructure and logistical support.

The challenges that come with refugee programs are profound. Refugees are often unwelcome in the country of sanctuary and have little or no voice in the host country government. The fear that the availability of services will draw even more refugees to the camps has led many host country governments (the US included) to design their camps like prisons, where the inhabitants are restricted from earning money, getting an education, or traveling freely.

Refugee camps sometimes double as military bases. This means they are, in effect, safe haven for soldiers, which often draws fire from the neighboring country. Finally, one of the real tragedies of refugee work is the simple fact that the weakest, who need the most help, are usually the least able to flee their country.

As an international refugee worker you will play a very important role that goes well beyond providing health care. In many situations, you can be the eyes of the international community, bringing the world's attention and support to the powerless ones caught in the middle of conflict.

3. *Giving shelter from the storm: disaster relief*

Disaster relief programs are implemented worldwide, in places that suffer destruction from natural disasters, such as floods, earthquakes, and hurricanes. Initially these programs focus on emergency care for the hurt and protection of those in harm's way. Long-term work is focused on rebuilding infrastructure so that infectious diseases can be prevented and the health care system can return to normal.

International response to natural disasters usually comes from governments and the large multilateral agencies that have financial and logistical resources to jump into action on a moment's notice, such as the International Committee of the Red Cross, or ICRC. However, international PVOs that are already in a country hit by a natural or man-made disaster can play an important role, by helping to mobilize international support.

As a disaster relief worker, you will face immense logistical challenges, not to mention questions about the usefulness of the donations, and the appropriate use of aid funds. These problems are not unique to disasters, but their impact is exacerbated by the urgent nature of emergency situations.

Disasters that occur in developing countries, where the resources of the health care system are already stretched or nonexistent, can often swamp the government's ability to coordinate the relief effort. The support that is sent in response to a disaster is often inappropriate, not driven by the needs at hand but rather by surplus supplies in the donor countries. When funds have been provided (the most versatile means of support), they have often been misused. Fortunately, since the early 1970s, the international community has become more adept at organizing and responding appropriately to these disasters.

4. Treating the sick: clinical care

In the past, the most common approach to international health was direct medical care, provided by a western doctor or nurse in a hospital, rural clinic, or refugee camp. The successors of these early approaches to international health continue today, for example in programs to treat cataracts, correct club feet or to remove giant hernias. Such clinical programs can make an enormous difference in individual lives.

Despite the continued popularity of this approach, however, over the last 30 years many have begun to question its efficiency and appropriateness. Reasons for reconsidering this approach include the limited number of patients that can be treated compared to the demand for treatment; the increase in the number of well-trained medical professionals in developing countries; and the recognition that western medical treatment seldom addresses the root causes of poor health.

If you are interested in providing direct care, you will probably find that the medically-based programs that have remained viable have evolved from an emphasis on direct care to one on training. Although many short-term volunteer programs still send doctors and nurses in for a week or two to run clinics, the focus is increasingly on building local clinical skills.

SIX TYPES OF GLOBAL HEALTH PROGRAMS
1. *Working with communities: primary health care*
2. *Setting up safe havens: refugee relief*
3. *Giving shelter from the storm: disaster relief*
4. *Treating the sick: clinical care*
5. *Sharing expertise: policy and program consultation*
6. *Finding a better way: research and training*

---

5. Sharing expertise: policy and program consultation

This is not exactly a program model like clinical or primary care. In this approach, consulting firms, multilateral agencies and PVOs work directly with developing country governments on their health care policies, building their capacity to design, administer, and finance health programs. Specific areas of assistance commonly include administration, biostatistics, epidemiology, research, policy design, evaluation and health care financing.

As a policy or program consultant, you can have a broad, sustainable impact on the health care delivery system in a developing country. You can focus on building local capacity within the limits of available resources.

A related approach works to change health policy from the other end of the political spectrum. International support is used to build the capacity of communities to organize and advocate for improved health care services from their own government. To be effective, both of these approaches require that the government be fairly stable, a tall order in many developing countries.

6. *Finding a better way: research and training*

Many US universities have established partnerships with peer institutions in developing countries. Such partnerships commonly involve exchange programs in which faculty and students can teach and attend courses, do joint research, and implement health programs. At their best, these programs build the networks and the skills of the future leaders in the health care field, in the US and overseas.

If you are a graduate student or faculty member of a US institution, there will be many opportunities for you to partner with academic colleagues overseas. You may not even need to be associated with a specific school if you are already in-country.

CYNTHIA MYNTTI
"Marginal people are the most interesting"

I really came to international health through the back door. As an undergraduate at the University of Utah, I got interested in the Middle East after meeting some graduate students from Palestine and Egypt. I was a misfit there, and so were they. I fell in love with them as people, emotionally and intellectually, and knew I wanted to go to the Middle East.

I went to Iran to teach right after I got my BA in political science in 1971. I arrived in Tehran in a miniskirt, and realized immediately how much I stood out. Of course what I didn't know was that most of the women around were wearing minis too, under their veils! In the Middle East, nothing is ever as it appears. That's what attracted me to it.

▲ ▲ ▲

I needed more training, so I got a master's degree in anthropology at American University in Beirut. I was interested in social development, but still not in health. After returning to the US, I had trouble finding a job, so I was encouraged to get a doctorate at the London School of Economics. I was fortunate to get funding to go to Yemen, to study population issues. Yemen is one of the least developed countries in the world, with an infant mortality rate at that time of over 200 babies per 1000 live births. The fertility rate was increasing, though, because women were beginning to breastfeed less. I went over to study this relationship between fertility and mortality.

For my PhD field work in anthropology, I lived in a Yemeni village for two years. There was no electricity and just a pail of water per week, that a neighbor would bring for me. I spent a lot of time talking to women. I was trying to learn about medicine in its social context: how people made decisions about health care. In those days, anthropologists were always talking about explanatory models, how an individual's view of the world determined his or her health-seeking behavior. My perspective was much more tied to politics and economics, on a household level.

Who in the family got to see a doctor if they were sick, and when, and why? When were women given access to care, and why?

▲ ▲ ▲

Because Yemen was less developed, it got lots of foreign aid funds. After finishing my field work, I was asked to do some consulting work for the German government, for USAID and for the UN Fund for Population Activities. These assignments supported the writing of my dissertation, which in turn led to a position with the Ford Foundation, as a program officer for the Middle East and North Africa. From my office in Cairo, I developed the Foundation's program in child and women's health.

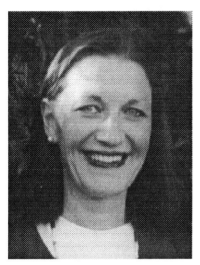

Cynthia researched womens' reproductive health programs in the Middle East.

I was remarkably autonomous in those days. I could find out who was doing interesting things and then see how best to support them. I was responsible for about $1 million in funds per year. The work was a privilege, and the responsibility was daunting!

What was nice about Ford was that there was a collegial dimension. We were encouraged to be modest: the local institution got the credit, not us. I got to support some wonderful programs, like the Traditional Medicine Research Institute, a group of Sudanese physicians who were interested in what they thought of as "folk medicine." I encouraged them to focus on how traditional medicine could be evaluated and integrated into public health practice. In Cairo I helped found a group called the Women's Health Book Collective. We decided to produce a kind of "Our Bodies, Ourselves" resource book, but for Middle Eastern women. So we had to deal with how the Egyptian censors would treat some of the material. It

*was a fascinating group of women: social workers and health profession-
als in veils and social scientists who were radical feminists. The book
finally came out in 1991.*

▲ ▲ ▲

*So I've been in international health both as an academic and a program
person, and I've found that one doesn't fit very easily into either world as
a result. It's a little uncomfortable. It's also true that I don't quite fit in
to any one place. My husband and I came back to Minnesota in 1993
because we didn't want to be expatriates forever, but I'm finding that no
one place in the world feels completely like home. We love it here, but I
keep getting interesting work offers overseas. Right now I'm spending
several months each spring in Beirut, as a visiting lecturer at the
American University. When I come home, I go out to the yard and start
gardening, no matter what the hour is. My neighbors have learned that
it's my way of coping with jet lag.*

*I guess maybe I have a more subtle appreciation of what home is. It used
to bother me to feel marginal, but I've come to think that marginal
people are the most interesting. Why not be marginal? The world is
collapsing around us, getting smaller all the time. Accept that discom-
fort. Recognize that it's okay, that you don't always have to fit in.*

*What other advice do I give students and people interested in going
overseas? Follow your passions. If it's a certain people, or a certain topic,
go with it. Get some field experience, say, in a grass roots organization,
not just academic training. That's critical for getting a real front-line feel
for what's happening. Learn to listen and to write well—those are
critical skills. You've got to be able to express yourself well. Practice and
find a good mentor.*

Editor's note: Since Cynthia was interviewed for the first edition of
this book, she has completed a masters' degree in architecture. She
is currently on a fellowship, studying housing systems in Finland.

CHAPTER THREE

What's In It For You?

Driven by the desire to help those less fortunate, the quest for adventure, or a myriad of other motivations, who hasn't fantasized about living the life of an expatriate?

Okay, maybe not everybody—but you have!

It takes a certain kind of person to give up many of the comforts of stateside life and take off for parts unknown. By reading this far, you've already begun to examine whether you are that kind of person. Your next step is to answer the most important question raised in this book: *Why do you want to go?*

It's a simple, yet crucial question, and one that's well worth spending time on. Identifying your personal goals in global health is the key to finding a satisfying position for yourself, whether that position is a once-in-a-lifetime volunteer assignment, or the beginning of a life-long career.

In this chapter, we will:

- look at many of the common motivations for going into global health;
- offer a dozen questions to help you hone your own goals; and
- give you a framework for writing out your goals and a description of your ideal position.

Why do they do it?

Why do thousands of health professionals decide every year to leave the comforts of home to work in some of the most difficult places in the world, under some of the most trying circumstances imaginable?

The motivations of global health workers are as varied as those who pursue the challenge. Below are some of the most common, along with a few caveats about each. As you read them, ask yourself: is this *my* motivation?

Altruism: Concern for the welfare of others remains one of the main reasons people decide to go into international health. It is often extremely altruistic work. However, making a substantial difference in people's lives is not easy. In many situations, it's not even possible. Many who are driven solely by the desire to "make things better" can become frustrated when they don't see immediate change.

Career advancement: Global health experience can be a real asset to your resume, even if you never go back overseas again. But some have found that once they've left their State-side work millieu for a while, they find it hard to fit back in. See Chapter Eight for more on readjusting to life in the US after working overseas.

Cutting edge work: Global health is a relatively new professional field, and one which is constantly evolving. The science is updated, new challenges pop up and new program approaches take center stage. While it can be a great opportunity if you are invigorated by change, it may be difficult if you're someone who looks for continuity and consistency in your professional life.

Adventure: The chance to live and work in exotic locations during times of war or disaster brings many into the field of international health for the sheer rush. Although the need for health care in these situations is very real, the people who specialize at working in them should be professionals with experience and training. Try to make sure you'll be up to the challenges you may encounter.

Cross-cultural experience: The chance to live and work in another country, with people of a different culture, is one of the great aspects of international health work. The experience can also enhance your skill at working in cross-cultural health care when you return to the

> **WHY PEOPLE CHOOSE TO WORK IN GLOBAL HEALTH**
> *Adventure:* I love a thrill.
> *Altruism:* The people need me.
> *Career advancement:* I need to get a better job.
> *Cutting edge work:* It's something new to think about.
> *Cross-cultural experience:* I can't wait to see the village market.
> *Money:* I think I'll make more.
> *Skill enhancement:* I want to learn tropical medicine.
> *Religion:* I'm on a mission from God.
> *Politics:* I'm on a mission from Che.
> *Escapism:* I gotta get outta here.
> *Personal growth:* I want to see if I can take it.
> *Learning experience:* It'll be good practice.
> *Retirement:* I don't play golf.

US. Of course, the flip side of immersion in a new environment is culture shock. See Chapter Seven on how to avoid the worst of it.

Money: (Whoa—wrong book!) Don't plan on getting rich in global health. Although your money will probably go further outside the US, and there are often added comforts to living overseas such as inexpensive house help, the overall pay is usually less than what you would make working in the health care system in the US. This is especially true when you're just starting out in a volunteer position with a small stipend, or working for a small organization.

Skill enhancement: Through work in international settings, many professionals—doctors who want to be administrators, nurses who want to become teachers—have been able to develop new skills. Working outside of your current job description is fine, but don't think that going overseas offers the opportunity to practice without the appropriate training and skills.

Religion: Religion is probably the oldest motivation for going overseas to provide health care. Many denominations have relief and development arms that are administered apart from their mission work. Others inextricably link development with the advancement of their religious beliefs. If you feel called to spread your religious beliefs, be totally honest and up front about your desire to prostelytize. Covert evangelizing has led to program expulsions and persecution of those involved (including local staff who usually don't have the luxury of leaving when the local government decides to clamp down.) If religion is important to you, there are plenty of organizations that do their missionary work openly—seek them out. (See the description in Chapter Five.)

Politics: If religion is the oldest reason for going overseas to help, then politics is probably the second. The concerns are the same, only more so. Know the politics of who's sending you, and of any groups you may encounter in-country. Before getting involved with a political group, be sure you are thoroughly clear on the safety implications of your choice, both for yourself and your colleagues.

Escapism: The desire to "get away" is a great reason for a vacation, not a career change. The reality is that global health is a profession that requires all the skills and training of other health careers, as well as the flexibity and energy to live and work in another country. It's no vacation.

Personal growth: It's perfectly okay to use a stint overseas as a way to test your mettle. But if you want to assess your interest before committing to advanced training or a long-term contract, a practice stint overseas is only one of many options. See Chapter Four for additional ideas on how to get that global experience.

Learning experience: Many students, especially in the health sciences, look at a global health opportunity as a good way to cap off their education. Unless you can be flexible about the kinds of work you'll do, as well as locations, timing, and finances, you may have trouble finding paying work, though educational opportunities overseas abound. See Chapter Five for more options.

Retirement: More and more people with experience and training in health care are volunteering to go overseas to work during their retirement. For example, about six percent of Peace Corps volunteers are over the age of 50. Older people may have more life skills and wisdom, as well as more credibility in traditional cultures, but health concerns may limit what you're willing to do.

Why do you want to do it?

The rewards of working in global health are tremendous—and so are the challenges. You'll need to be very clear about what you're trying to accomplish. The following questions will help you set your goals and describe your ideal position.

1. Is global health going to be my career or an avocation?

While more and more people are looking at international health as a life-long career, many find creative ways of mixing overseas work with Stateside careers and families. Frequent flier programs, the internet, early retirement, and sabbaticals have all helped to make international health work possible for those who can't stay overseas for long periods.

2. When is the right time in my life to go overseas?

While most people involved in international health are in their twenties and thirties, other age groups are increasingly getting involved. Many are using midcareer sabbaticals, annual vacations, and retirement as opportunities to work overseas. Obviously though, the more family obligations, job constraints and mortgages you have, the less flexibility you enjoy.

3. How soon can I go?

Here is where you may encounter a frustrating reality of the international health job market. The level of competition, the fluidity in staffing, and the time and money it takes for organizations to place people in the field all make flexibility key for getting the best jobs. Don't expect an organization to build a job around your one-week summer vacation, unless you've got unique technical skills they need or you are willing to cover your own expenses, and then some.

By the same token, being able to leave on a moment's notice when the need arises can help you land a great position. Try to be ready to go when they call. See Chapters Six and Seven on preparation. The earlier you can start to plan your availability, the better.

4. How long can I be gone?

How long can you be away from job, family, house, garden, goldfish? Can you stand to miss the first-run movie premieres? Here's reality check number two: generally, the longer you can commit, the better your chances of landing a job. Because it usually takes up to six months from the time a position is posted until the new hire arrives in the field and becomes a productive part of the project, most organizations won't send people over for less than a

A CHECKLIST: WHAT'S ON YOUR RESUME?

teaching expertise
cross cultural experience
knowledge of infectious diseases
family planning expertise
vaccine preventable illnesses
nutrition background
management of childhood illness
organizational development
needs assessment training
program planning expertise
administrative ability
evaluation experience
grant writing successes
health education
training in epidemiology
biostatistics skill
financial management
supervisory experience
volunteer work
second or third language

year. The vast majority will require two-or three-year commitments.

While there are some opportunities for going overseas to work for short periods, these are usually either consultancies for highly experienced professionals, or work-study tours that require you to cover your expenses.

5. What types of work can I do?

Flexibility is key, not only to getting a position but also enjoying the work. It's impossible to write a job description that covers all that you might be called upon to do in the field. One day you'll be at an inter-agency coordinating meeting in a hospital board room, and the next day you'll be training village health workers under a tree. A day later, you could be fixing a flat on a dirt road.

ASK YOURSELF
Is global health a career or an avocation?
When is the right time to go overseas?
How soon can I go?
How long can I be gone?
What types of work can I do?
Do I need more training?
Where do I want to go?
Should I learn another language?
How important is personal security to me?
How about those creature comforts?
Is my family coming along?
How much money must I make overseas?

The definition of global health work is expanding all the time. Are you qualified? How much do you know about training, curriculum development, tropical medicine, intervention areas (infectious diseases, family planning, immunization programs, nutrition, integrated management of childhood illness), as well as organizational development, needs assessment, program planning, administration, evaluation, grant writing/fundraising, health information systems, epidemiology, biostatistics, financial management, staff supervision, or community development? The more of these areas you can master, the more employable you'll be.

6. Do I need more training?

Thirty years ago, all you needed was medical training, a plane ticket, passport, and a really good pair of boots. Today most people entering global health as a career or a serious avocation have a master's degree in public health (MPH). This is a degree that can provide the basic skills needed to start in field work. In addition to the obvious specialization in international health, useful areas of training within public health include epidemiology, maternal and child health, health education and administration (See the box on the previous page for a longer list).

As the number of people entering the field has grown, more folks are investing in a PhD, especially for the long-term, high-end jobs. Be forewarned: academic global health programs are competitive. If you can't invest in a full-time program, there are other shorter (or long-distance) options at good schools, such as London School of Hygiene and Tropical Medicine, Boston University and Johns Hopkins.

7. Where do I want to work?

If you are just finishing an Arabic immersion program, you are probably going to want to focus on the Middle East or North Africa. While this will help you narrow your job search, it will also limit your options. If you're willing to go where the winds take you, many more options will open up. Many seasoned global health workers have developed technical skills or areas of expertise such as refugee relief work, that are transferable from country to country.

8. Should I learn another language?

Obviously, this depends on where you'll be. You can get by in many countries speaking English, but knowing the language gives you greater credibility and a better understanding of the local culture. Once you've signed up for that first assignment, language immersion programs and hiring a local tutor in-country are highly recommended, even for very short assignments or trips.

What language is most useful? Again, it depends on your geographic preferences. Many people looking at a career in international work go for Spanish (Latin America), Arabic (the Middle East and North Africa), or French (west Africa and former Indochina).

If you simply have a tin ear, keep trying to learn at least a few words. You'll be viewed much more favorably if you can thank people in their own language, even if you massacre the syntax and grammar. On the other hand, you may be able to avoid the language issue altogether, either by focusing on shorter term emergency disaster and refugee work, or by developing a specific transferable specialty.

9. How important is personal security to me and those I'm taking along?

International health sometimes attracts adrenaline junkies—people who are invigorated by chaos, uncertainty and danger. Sadly, with all the stories of terrorism and violence in the news, there seem to be more and more places that can provide that kind of rush. Even if you are going to a more sedate place, personal security should be considered.

Can you live without easy access to a doctor? How do you feel about men with guns, cars without seatbelts, or hospitals without blood banks? If it's hard for you to contemplate injustice, how will you react when you witness it personally? Will your reaction endanger you or your colleagues? (For the U.S. State Department's perspective on where you'll be safest, you can check on the latest security concerns by country, at travel.state.gov/travel.)

10. How about those creature comforts?

Are you the type that chafes at airport delays, needs a toilet seat, or shudders at the thought of rice and beans every day for a year? Needless to say, you are probably not cut out for some types of global health work. It's wise to be realistic about this one: no sense making yourself miserable by agreeing to an assignment in the outback, when you'd really be much more effective in the home office.

11. Is my family coming along?

Except for long term, salaried positions that usually go to career professionals, few global health jobs will cover the expense of sending the family along. (Some fellowship programs may pay for a dependent or two. Or you may have a talented spouse who can transfer his/her skills overseas.)

Weigh the cost of a whole-family move carefully: Raising children overseas can be a mixed bag. On the down side you have security, health care, education, and expense of transport to consider. On the plus side, your kids may learn another language and see firsthand how the vast majority of the world's children live—an experience they will never forget. See Chapters Seven and Eight for a bit more on family considerations.

12. How much money must I make while overseas?

In general, the likelihood of making money is directly related to the extent of your experience. University and charitable short term work-study programs usually require you to cover at least a portion of your own costs (transport, visas, health insurance, food, etc.). Many programs set you up with local host families. These programs are a good way to get your feet wet, if you can afford them.

"Volunteer" positions are those for no pay or stipend pay, and include the Peace Corps and many voluntary or religious organizations. These groups provide overseas opportunities to those with training and limited experience. Covered costs may include transport to and from; in-country housing (usually communal and always low end); health and medivac insurance; immunizations and visa fees. Think of these as break-even opportunities.

Salaried positions are mostly long-term. Salaries range from stipends to pay as generous as anything you'll find in the US. This is all discussed in greater detail in Chapter Five.

DAVID NEWBERRY
"You have to find your motivation"

My motivation for global health service probably goes back to my experience during the Korean War where I saw the desperate needs of a poverty-stricken people in a conflict situation. My life was mysteriously saved more than once during that campaign, so I always felt that there was a purpose for my life that I had better try to carry out.

Being of Native American descent, there were challenges in my life, such as my father's premature death, which had to be dealt with and overcome before moving on to achieve the potential for working with others. Leaving the world a better place to live in is the Indian philosophy.

Rejoining society following the Korean War it was obvious that helping others required qualifications and preparation. I entered a Quaker College as a pre-med student, often challenging their gentle beliefs and presenting a counter-challenge as a militant person in a non-violent philosophical and religious community.

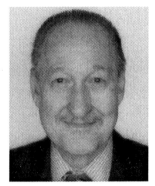

David: Seeds for international service planted during the Korean War.

After college, I did some graduate training and was employed by a medical research group. My job was to prepare everything needed in using animal subjects for some early liver transplant studies

Epidemiology was always of high interest, and is even more so now! This interest prompted me to join the Centers for Disease Control in 1964, as a venereal disease epidemiologist assigned to the New York City team. Working out of the Fort Greene Social Hygiene Clinic in Brooklyn opened a whole new world. Here was a kid from South and Midwest being paid to interview people about their sex lives!

Later I was assigned by CDC to Memphis, Shelby County Tuberculosis

Division as the acting director. We had about 2000 cases on the books. The West Tennessee Chest Hospital was just across the street, which served as a rotation experience for senior medical students. We had one deceased patient who exposed three medical students to tuberculosis during her autopsy. All three became infected! This CDC assignment provided me with incredible experience in managing the clinical and social aspects of an infectious disease.

CDC selected me and my family to work in the Smallpox Eradication and Measles Control program in West Africa. Before this assignment I completed the CDC Epidemic Intelligence Service (EIS) training in 1968. My assignment was in the west African country of Ghana as the Chief of Party for smallpox eradication.

Later CDC assigned me to Nigeria conducting a disease and demographic survey in northern Nigeria. There I learned to truly appreciate the Housa-Fulani ethnic group. This experience really touched my life. Learning the language and just a bit of their culture was one of the most important parts of my international career. I learned there are many cultural values and practices not easily accepted by outsiders. For example, as a 70 year old person today, I can go into any Housa-Fulani house and out of courtesy they would have to listen to what I had to say, unless, ofcourse, there was an octogenarian present! Traditional views are very powerful and when tradition and and culture and science collide - science will always lose.

On my way back from Nigeria, I was intercepted at the airport and informed that Vietnam had fallen to the communists and that thousands of refugees would be entering the US. CDC sent me with a cadre of three to Fort Chaffee, Arkansas to set up infectious disease screening and immunization services for refugees. My wife and children had remained in Nigeria until the school semester ended. Meanwhile in Fort Chaffee, the population of that place went from about 12 personnel to a city of 30,000 in a matter of about 15 days. The US Army called this activity "Operation New Life." It was a most moving experience and one that changed my family forever. When my wife and children arrived from Nigeria, I met the plane and informed her, "I have located a house for us to live in. The better news is that we have increased our family with a

Vietnamese refugee family." This family consisted of husband, wife and seven children. We had five surviving children out of six, and we later legally adopted the mother of the Vietnamese family. Again we learned to live among members of another culture and we learned to appreciate their traditions. It has been a wonderful experience.

During my 25 year tenure at the Centers for Disease Control and Prevention I never had a day that I felt bored or "burned out"! Every day was a new adventure at CDC. I was assigned to a number of short term assignments in Southeast Asia and in Africa. In 1986 I retired from the CDC and went to work for the Carter Center in the guinea worm eradication program in Ghana. I set up the original program there in 1988. That program really drove the point home that one must understand the culture before any progress can be made. The epidemiologist's nightmare is trying to achieve an eradication goal by changing human behavior against cultural norms. One must be innovative in these circumstances.

In one area, where eight villages shared a single surface water source, guinea worm was out of control. I met one man who had 25 guinea worms at the same time. He suffered horribly. People infected with guinea worm in those villages would soothe their sores in the water to relieve their pain. But in the process the worm would release millions of larvae into the water for others to become infected. The release of the guinea worm larva is how the agent spread to all eight villages.

The chiefs of the eight villages, who understood the transmission process, wanted me to solve the problem of water access because none of them had control of villagers from any village but thier own. My only suggestion was to add to their Housa greeting the phrase, "have you filtered your water through a cloth today?" One has to appreciate Housa greetings, which are lengthy and complex but rooted in health. Hausas will greet by first asking about your spouse, children and so forth.

A few months after my talk with the chiefs of the eight villages, one of my volunteer Ghanaian workers went up to visit the area and to assess the water control measures. He returned and reported that the chiefs had solved their water control problem and a guard was posted to fine on-

*the-spot those who went into the water with sores. The observer was
amazed to also report that wherever he went he was greeted with "How
is your wife, how are your children and have you filtered your water
today?"*

*Starting at CARE USA about 10 years ago was my first long term PVO
experience. My role was Senior Advisor for Children's Health. We
worked on training community health workers (CHWs) to assess,
classify, treat and prevent malaria, diarrhea and pneumonia. The
CHWs were all female. Through good training and better clinical
practical sessions, which emphasized direct application of clinical
proficiency and not just "book learning," these workers are incredible
and effective. In two years with ongoing, clinic-based training these
ladies reduced under-five mortality by 50%.*

*Five years ago, I started on my third eradication program, the eradica-
tion of polio. My current job is to serve as the project director for the
CORE Group Partners polio eradication project. When you say those
magic words "eradication program", you will have my undivided
attention.*

*So, I've been blessed with a varied career. It is not clear to me what to
tell those seeking a lifetime of service to the poorest of the poor, but I
doknow that you must have enthusiasm and lots of passion for what you
are doing. Agencies are more likely to be attracted to your enthusiasm in
conjunction with experience and qualifications. Identify the people and
institutions that you are attracted to, and pursue them with enthusiasm.
Find where you can be of service. But do remember that you should be
doing what provides you with personal and professional satisfaction and
please, don't take a job just for money.*

*Lastly, keep your focus on motivation. On my office wall is a photograph
of a lovely, healthy African mother, nursing her obviously health
baby. The baby is beautiful and the mother is glowing. When I get
discouraged, I look at that mom, it makes me realize and appreciate
what I am all about and why I am here.*

CHAPTER FOUR

Must You Leave Home?

If you don't have the money to get a master's degree in international health nor the time to do a Peace Corps stint, but you want to test your interest in global health, this chapter is for you.

In this chapter you'll learn about options that require less time or money, and ways you can experience the day-to-day realities of working in global health.

The value of building a broad network of contacts is stressed throughout this book, beginning in this chapter. Although a rapidly growing discipline, global health is still a pretty small arena. *Who* you know is often just as important as what you know. Connections and reputation are crucial to success in getting a job, and especially important in establishing a career in international health. The more people you know, working in more places, the better.

Anyway, as you are meeting people and making decisions

about entering the field of global health, here are nine options for getting your feet wet. The list can be expanded to the bounds of your imagination and your own goals.

Ten ways to get your feet wet

1. Talk to past volunteers.

This work changes people. Everyone comes back with a set of experiences to tell and most love the opportunity to talk. A few hours at the local tap room or coffee house can be extremely enlightening and entertaining. Where did you work? What did you do? Who did you work with? What was it like? If you want to get serious, Chapter Six gives you a pretty exhaustive list of questions to ask.

2. Join international health groups.

The Global Health Council's Global Health Action Network is a good place to start. A national program that mobilizes support for global health in the developing world, provides its members

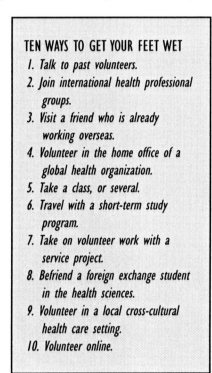

TEN WAYS TO GET YOUR FEET WET
1. Talk to past volunteers.
2. Join international health professional groups.
3. Visit a friend who is already working overseas.
4. Volunteer in the home office of a global health organization.
5. Take a class, or several.
6. Travel with a short-term study program.
7. Take on volunteer work with a service project.
8. Befriend a foreign exchange student in the health sciences.
9. Volunteer in a local cross-cultural health care setting.
10. Volunteer online.

with the resources and tools to communicate with elected officials and others about urgent global health matters, including maternal and child health, HIV/AIDS, and infectious disease. Volunteer advocates must be willing to support the Council's positions on specific international health policies that relate to one of its five focus areas: child survival; maternal health and survival; reproductive health and family planning; HIV/AIDS; and infectious disease. You can learn more by checking the Council's website, at www.globalhealth.org.

There are also lots of local internationally-oriented organizations that occasionally focus on health care issues. These organizations can often be found in your community through word of mouth, as they often work together. Talk to people at your church, fraternal organization or school to see if they are supporting any overseas projects.

3. Visit a friend who is already working overseas.

Got a week or two of vacation coming up and no place to go? This is an excellent way to get an intimate view of global health. Most field projects are used to having visitors, including home office staff, volunteers, funders and evaluators. While this can disrupt program work (the real reason they're all out there in the first place), visitors who aren't pushy and don't expect extra amenities are usually welcome.

A good way to grease the skids is to offer to take mail—going and coming. Give plenty of warning about your arrival. If you can't go, be an e-mail pen pal to your friend. Most projects now have at least sporadic internet access. You can learn a lot that way.

4. Volunteer in the home office of a US-based global health organization.

At last count, there were over 1,000 US-based organizations involved in international health. While many are on the coasts, almost every US city is home to at least some kind of world friendship organization where you can volunteer. This is an excellent way to build up connections with practitioners, to learn the workings of global health from the home office perspective, and to be closer to where the jobs are.

There is even competition for this volunteer work. Organizations get phone calls every day from people who want to get involved. Those who get their foot in the door are willing to help out on anything whenever it's needed, from stuffing envelopes to housing overseas volunteers while they're in town.

Since 1979, over one hundred mutual assistance associations (MAAs) have been established throughout the US. These nonprofit social service organizations are run by and for immigrant communities. Some of these organizations have attempted to reestablish ties with their homeland and do development work. These could easily benefit from volunteer input.

5. Take a class, or several.

In the US there are many schools of public health, medicine and international development with significant international health offerings. Most universities will offer at least one course that covers global health or international development. Be creative—check the education department for international development education, for example.

Many schools with health science programs also have a campus international health committee of some kind. Some schools, such as Boston University and Johns

Hopkins University, have abbreviated programs where you can take intensive course work in an area of international health for two to three months.

A good academic international health program attracts students from a variety of countries who bring their backgrounds and expertise to the course. Take the time to meet them outside of class. You might get a chance to partner with them in their home country some day.

6. Travel with a short-term study program.

Many universities, PVOs, religious institutions, and advocacy groups offer short-term (one week to six months) study sessions in developing countries. This is an excellent way to get a first-hand view of international health and development programs. Check the Global Health Council web site, (www globalhealthcouncil.org) for listings.

Through such programs, you can often see community-based health facilities, rural clinics, ministry of health offices, international PVOs and city hospitals. Study tours also give you a chance to meet with a variety of health professionals, both nationals and internationals, as well as students. You usually pay all of your own expenses.

Be forewarned: while these programs are an excellent opportunity to get a quick view of what you could be doing as a global health worker, in the eyes of most potential employers, they don't count as a first overseas assignment.

7. Take on volunteer work with a service project.

Many colleges and universities, as well as church groups offer service learning opportunities. In contrast to study programs, short-term "service vacations" tend to focus more on a community experience and less on abstract learning about the health care system.

In such programs, you live and work with community members on a project such as building latrines or teaching community health workers. Some work programs are more specialized, such as Operation Smile, an agency which sends volunteer surgeons abroad to perform reconstructive surgeries. The costs of the trip are often shared among the participant, the organization and the community. Many programs arrange for your housing with a local family.

If you are really adventurous, but too young to apply for a college program or job, you may want to investigate high school programs that let you try out global health work for several weeks. One such organization is Amigos de Las Americas, which places young adults in Peace Corps-like assignments for four to six weeks at a time. Read Maria Witt's account of her Amigos stint, following this chapter.

8. Befriend an exchange student in the health sciences.
Every year, thousands of foreign health science students come to the US for training. If you live in a university or college town, helping out with housing, tutoring or just getting around town can lead to a life-long friendship. It is also another avenue for learning about global health. Stay connected when your pal returns home, through the internet, the mail and the phone.

9. Volunteer or work in a local cross-cultural health care setting.
You don't have to travel overseas to work in international health. Over the past 50 years there has been a major change in the cultural complexion of the United States, with the

influx of the greatest wave of immigrants since the 1880s. Recently arriving refugees and immigrants from Southeast Asia, Africa, Eastern Europe and Latin America have brought their own languages and cultural beliefs, many of which have challenged the US health care system.

Not all US immigrants are poor, of course, but many are. So are people in many non-immigrant groups. The experience of working with migrant workers in Florida, American Indians on reservations in Arizona, or coal miners in Appalachia can be excellent training for working with poor people overseas. Not to mention the possibility of improving life for those close to home!

10. Volunteer online.

Thanks to the internet, you don't even have to leave the comfort of your own home to build international health experience. A new program through United Nations Volunteers, called Online Volunteers, links individuals with useful skills to field programs in developing countries. Volunteers are needed to help translate documents, write articles or reports, do research, build web sites or mentor young people. More information is on the program's website, www.onlinevolunteering.org.

MARIA WITT
"I know the path I want"

I spent two years in Mexico when I was about nine years old, when my parents moved our family to Cuernavaca, so I speak pretty good Spanish. But the first time I went overseas by myself was in the summer after tenth grade, when I was 16. I went with a program called Amigos de las Americas, which is designed to give young adults an international service experience. I heard about it from the brother of a friend of mine. You go with a partner to a village and work for eight weeks or so, doing basic public health or education projects.

The Amigos program is divided into chapters, by location. Our chapter met every other week for six months. We got lots of training, and we had to raise the money to go, about $3,500. Some of the money went to pay for our trip and room and board, but most of it goes to pay for supplies for the projects we helped with. I sold fruit and wrote fundraising letters to family members and friends to get the money. My parents helped with some, too.

As a high school student, Maria taught rural kids in Honduras about hygiene.

I went to Honduras in 1996, and liked the experience so much that I went back the following year to the Dominican Republic. Now, in the summer after my freshman year at college, I'll be going to Guanajuato, Mexico, to be an Amigos supervisor. I'll be responsible for volunteers like myself, in four different towns. I'm looking forward to it.

▲ ▲ ▲

I've had a pretty middle class, urban life style. Even though we live in a neighborhood in Washington DC which is full of Latinos, there was a huge difference between them and the people in the villages where I lived, some of whom had never even left their towns. I wanted to try something completely different, as far from my current experience as possible.

My parents thought it was a good idea, at least in theory. They were excited about me going, but they had some problems with me being alone in a small town with only one other American girl. There were a lot of issues that they could just sit around daydreaming about, like what if I would break my leg, what if something happened. I wouldn't get the treatment I would get here.

The towns I was in were so rural that there was no fast way out. In the Dominican Republic, there was literally no way out of town by car. One truck came once a week to bring supplies and some food. It was an hour's walk through scrubby woods to get to the nearest town.

When I got there that concerned me, but at that point there really wasn't anything I could do about it. I figured out that being safe has a lot to do with how you carry yourself. You have to think about how to prevent dangerous situations. I had been prepared through my training for potentially tricky situations and how to deal with them. Also, Amigos has rules about how to dress. They tell you to think of yourself as a public health worker, not as an exchange student, or a tourist, and to dress and act accordingly.

In terms of health safety, you have to realize that you are in a Third World country, and that the health care will not be the same as in the United States. However, people in the town have lived there for their whole lives and have dealt with many problems. If you broke your leg, they would be able to find a way for you to get to a medical center. Once I realized this, I was able to relax more.

▲ ▲ ▲

In Honduras, I did community sanitation projects; mainly building latrines. We built six latrines, with materials we had raised money for. We had cement toilet bowls, and plastic tubing, to make a simple toilet that you could flush with a bucket. But that didn't take all of our time, and we were expected to figure out what else to do, based on what the townspeople wanted. So we did a worm project. There are special kinds of worms that make fertilizers out of animal manure. They also reproduce really quickly, so people could give a few worms to their neighbors to start another box and make more fertilizer.

In the Dominican Republic, I also did community sanitation, but people had a little more money, and some people already had latrines. Our work was mainly organizing and motivating the town, along with implementing other concurrent projects. We worked on planting gardens with seeds we brought along. We also gave talks in the schools, playing with kids and teaching about basic hygiene and the environment. We talked about trash pickup, toothbrushing and nutrition. We also spent a lot of time getting to know our host family and community, talking, playing cards or even helping to sort beans.

▲ ▲ ▲

Even though both places were really tiny towns, I wasn't bored at all. We ate with seven different families. Each day we worked with the family that was feeding us. There were times when I was frustrated, because I didn't understand what was going on. There were times that I felt I had offended someone without having any idea how. It was also frustrating to realize that no matter how kind people were, we were never going to really be a part of the community. We made amazing connections and had wonderful relationships, but this never changed the fact that our backgrounds were so different.

I don't know how much I helped to improve the health of the small villages where I stayed, in that short a time. But some kids in the villages where we were now know about toothbrushing, and we were able to show people some technical shortcuts for making latrines. But that isn't the biggest focus. It definitely made an impact just to be there, just to be *paying attention to what was going on. Our goal wasn't to change lives in our two-month stay. Rather, we wanted to increase awareness in these communities about health issues as well as change negative perceptions they may have had about North Americans.*

▲ ▲ ▲

My work with Amigos has been something that I've only done in the summer, but I think about it all the time. My college classes all seem to relate, too. Like in an education class, we read the theories of Paolo Freire, and it made me think about different ways of teaching people to read, or about health issues.

There are few things I've done in my life for only two months that I can honestly say changed me completely; my focus, my goals and my outlook on life. I'll probably have something to do with community organizing or public health when I graduate. I'm just starting on my path, but because of what I've done already, I know this is the way I want to go.

Editor's note: Since she was interviewed for the first edition of this book, Maria has graduated from Brown University and worked as a labor and political organizer. She continues to travel outside the US as often as possible.

Amigos de las Americas is an international, voluntary, nongovernmental, not-for-profit organization that, through service, provides leadership development opportunities for young people; promotes community health in Latin America; and facilitates cross-cultural understanding for the people of the Americas. For more information, check the Amigos web site: www.amigoslink.org

CHAPTER FIVE

Who's Hiring?

In the US alone, there are over 1000 organizations involved in global health. With so many organizations to choose among, how will you know which is best for you? The trick is to start with yourself. Now might be a good time to review your answers to the questions in Chapter Three, to refocus on what your needs are and what you hope to achieve. This will help you narrow down your search for the organization that will provide the right fit.

Once you start looking at global health organizations, you'll need a way to keep from being overwhelmed. One way to organize your thoughts is to focus on the *types* of organizations. As we see it, there are several basic types of global health groups. Knowing what they are, and what they are looking for in employees and volunteers is important —even if, in the end, you choose *not* to work within an established outfit.

In this chapter, we'll take a more detailed look at these types of organizations. We begin with those that often serve as career entry points, and work our way up to the big-time, big-money groups. We'll also look at some non-traditional approaches you may want to consider.

Types of global health groups

1. Peace Corps

Here's one organization that's in a category of its own. The United States Peace Corps has long been one of the best ways to get that coveted first overseas experience. Even business majors are now applying to the Peace Corps as a way to get international exposure. They may have a point: many job recruiters with other international health organizations view a Peace Corps stint on your resume as evidence of your ability to live and work overseas without self-destructing.

Each Peace Corps volunteer (or PCV) is placed with a host country non-governmental organization (NGO) or local government agency. Health projects usually focus on sustainable health education, training, and community organizing.

Peace Corps is looking both for individuals with specific technical skills (i.e., nursing or public health) and those from a liberal arts background with strong organizational leadership skills and experience. Each PCV receives three months of training prior to service in the field. This includes job skills training as well as Peace Corps' excellent language training.

The lifestyle for a PCV varies greatly from one country to another. You may live in a mud hut in rural Africa, in a modern apartment building in eastern Europe, or anywhere in between. In addition to housing, volunteers receive a living stipend, health care coverage and vacation time during their field experience and round trip travel to and from the assignment. After completing an assignment, PCVs receive an adjustment allowance for each month successfully completed, graduate school opportunities through the Masters International Program and Fellows USA program, and noncompetitive eligibility status when applying for federal jobs. Many PCVs have also been able to arrange for deferrals of student loans during an assignment; however Peace Corps does not guarantee this.

While there is no assurance that you will go to the country of your choosing, Peace Corps recruiters will work with you to identify an assignment that fits your skills, educational background and experience. Language skills, date of availability and medical history are also considered. Flexibility about where you end up is the key.

Peace Corps is one of the biggest players in global health employment, receiving about 10,000 applications each year (for all types of work, not just health.) It has just over 7,500 volunteers in the field. The average age of those placed is 28, but more than five percent are over 50. Married couples are welcome, but children are not.

The basic requirements are two-fold: the minimal standard set by the US Congress (US citizenship, 18 years or older, and good health) and those established by the host country government. Because all Peace Corps projects are implemented at the invitation of the host country, requirements are often added, including technical expertise and college degrees. Ninety five percent of all Peace Corps volunteers have at least a bachelor's degree.

Peace Corps offices are located in most large cities throughout the US and are listed in the US government section of the yellow pages directory. The Peace Corps can also be found on the internet at ww.peacecorps.org. The Corps has a large recruitment program involving returned volunteers. Check Huy Pham's profile following Chapter Seven, for one take on a Peace Corps assignment.

2. Smaller Private Voluntary Organizations (PVOs)

Smaller PVOs are a good next step for returning Peace Corps volunteers or someone seeking entry-level work. If you can work out the timing and meet their other requirements, they can also be a good first assignment. The smaller PVOs are the most numerous and most heterogeneous type of organizations in this list, with the most varied missions, approaches to global health, and organizational cultures.

In addition to their size, they share a common organizational structure as private tax-exempt corporations and tend to be volunteer-based with relatively small home office staffs. Many focus their programs in a particular country (i.e. Salvadoran American Health Foundation, or Medical Outreach for Armenians). Others specialize in an area of technical expertise (i.e. American Leprosy Foundation and American Dentists for Foreign Service).

The smaller PVOs generally can offer broad flexibility in their positions, with the opportunity to learn new skills. Sounds great, but it can lead to a harrowing work life. What many such organizations lack in structure, financial stability, and detailed job descriptions, they make up for in unpaid overtime. But if you have a gung ho attitude, and the willingness to pay your dues, you can grow into a good position quickly. Cheryl Robertson, profiled after Chapter One, has worked for many years with two small PVOs.

Organizations in this category are usually looking for generalists with strong people and organizational skills. If the agency specializes in a technical area, they'll be snapping up well-trained practitioners. Most positions require one to three years of overseas work experience and relevant graduate school education. They often want people to commit to at least one year. Language fluency may be required in Spanish, French and Arabic-speaking countries. In other countries, it's easier to get in without knowing the language because of the limited pool of qualified job candidates.

The compensation tends to be on the low side, with the agency often providing international transport, a basic living stipend, housing with local families or communal housing with other volunteers, and medical evacuation insurance. Before you sign on with a PVO, be sure to check the lists of questions in Chapters Six and Seven.

A note on communal living: After returning from a difficult tour working in an East African refugee camp for six months, one former PVO staffer said the most difficult aspect was living with the other Americans!

Smaller PVOs use a variety of methods to recruit volunteers and staff. The network among many of the PVOs is pretty tight, with organizations sharing resumes and talking about candidates all the time. Jobs are also posted in the more common job placement publications (see the back of the book for a listing), at national conferences (Global Health Council and American Public Health Association especially) and on organizational websites.

Getting your foot in the door of a small PVO requires creativity and persistence. A great way is to volunteer in a home office. Some volunteers have developed long-term relationships with organizations and gone overseas repeatedly for shorter periods, or even shared a position with field staff. This way they've been able to enjoy the challenges of working overseas without having to forgo the perks of US life.

Unless you live in New York, Washington or Los Angeles, finding small PVOs in your community can be a challenge. Your best bet is to buy the latest edition of the Global Health Council's *Global Health Directory,* available from their website, www.globalhealthcouncil.org.

3. United Nations Volunteers (UNV)

Here's another volunteer organization that's a category in itself. The United Nations Volunteers (UNV) was formed in 1970 as part of the United Nations Development Program. UN Volunteers are placed in UN-member countries to work in partnership with local governments, UN agencies, development banks, and private voluntary and nongovernmental organizations in health care and other development-related professions.

Currently there are over 4,000 UN Volunteers from 150 countries, working *in* 130 countries. The work is varied, but focuses on technical cooperation with local governments, community-based initiatives for self-reliance, humanitarian relief and rehabilitation, support of elections and peace building.

The requirements for getting a position are academic training, several years of relevant work experience, commitment to serving others, readiness to work in difficult conditions, and the ability to listen and work with people from a variety of cultures. Compared to the Peace Corps, UNV is more competitive, more professionalized, and a better bet for someone with some overseas health experience than for a newcomer to the field. You must be at least 25 to apply.

As a UN Volunteer you receive a "settling in grant" at the beginning of your assignment, a monthly living allowance to cover expenses, travel to and from the worksite, life/health and disability insurance, annual leave and a resettlement allowance after you complete your assignment.

You can apply on line, and your application will be placed in a roster for up to two years. You will be contacted when a suitable position turns up.

The primary benefits of UNV work are the chance to work with a multinational group in a developing country, the prestige of working for the UN, and the in-country administrative and technical support. Further information on the UNV and its application process is available on their website, www.unv.org.

4. Large Private Voluntary Organizations (PVOs)

These are the organizations most of us think of when we hear the words "global health"—Save the Children, CARE, Oxfam, Project Hope, the International Committee of the Red Cross. Compared to their smaller counterparts, the agencies in this category tend to be older and more established. Like their smaller cousins, most big PVOs are nonprofit corporations, supported by public and private sources. Many, such as Catholic Relief Services or Lutheran World Relief, are supported by religious organizations.

Where many of the smaller PVOs may be "personality-driven," molded by the vision (or whim) of a founder, these larger organizations tend to be policy-driven. As older organizations, they have survived the manic development and growth phase that most nonprofit organizations go through in their first years. Most are now on-going, stable concerns, with professional administrators, multi-million dollar budgets, and programs around the world. The larger PVOs often work in several sectors besides health care, including economic development, disaster relief, agriculture, or human rights.

In general, working for a larger PVO gives you the opportunity to focus on your technical specialty, relieving you of the administrative hassles that can bedevil your counterparts in smaller organizations. Setting up personnel benefits, buying airline tickets and retrieving lost luggage, or reviewing monthly financial reports can all fall under someone else's job description.

Assuming that you've developed the necessary skills and have the required experience, you can focus on your *real* work: designing the program evaluation, carrying out the anti-malaria intervention campaign, writing the training curriculum. For one view of work with a large PVO, read Huy Pham's profile following Chapter Seven.

The larger PVOs hire a wide variety of workers, including short-term consultants with specialized expertise, long-term project directors with strong administrative experience, and medium-term line staff. Three to five years of previous overseas experience, graduate school training, language fluency, and specialized technical skills (survey techniques, rapid rural appraisal, accounting, etc.) are common requirements. Your competition won't be limited to fellow expatriates.

Appropriately, many PVOs prefer to place host country nationals in leadership positions.

The best way to approach the larger PVOs is through your network of contacts and applying to posted positions. However, most of the large PVOs also have databases, so even sending in an unsolicited resume can be helpful if your experience and training fit the organization's needs. See more on this in the section on resumes, in Chapter Six.

The recruitment process of larger PVOs is similar to that of smaller ones, except you will probably be dealing with a person in human resources rather than your future supervisor, at least initially. Most positions offer candidates better salaries and benefits than you would receive with the smaller organizations, often including housing allowances, transportation of personal goods, and paid home leaves.

Most of the larger PVOs have large in-country offices in the capital city. In addition, many larger PVOs will often have regional offices that provide administrative and technical support to their field programs. The international development "revolving door" has allowed many who stay with the same organization for extended periods to divide their lives between home office and field assignments.

5. Consulting Firms

John Snow, Inc., Management Sciences for Health, and Development Associates— you might not recognize their names, but these are the giants among the many consulting firms which have made an impact in global health in the past 30 years. Unlike the organizations we've looked at so far, the agencies in this category are run like for-profit businesses (though strictly speaking, some are non-profits.)

Consulting firms work under contract with government and multilateral agencies worldwide. Most of their work tends to be at the policy level, interacting with senior government and private sector types, rather than with community members. Many have established in-country affiliate organizations, which provide direct services.

The qualifications for employment are usually quite stiff, with language requirements, graduate degrees up to post doctoral training, and five to ten years of relevant overseas experience. Many people enjoy the work as it can provide a lot of variety, as well as the opportunity to live primarily in the US and travel overseas on short-term assignments.

Not many entry level overseas options here, unless you boast special expertise or academic training. But the home offices of these firms are classic entry points for public health and international development graduates. Bert Hirschhorn, profiled after this chapter, built much of his overseas career through sequential assignments for consulting firms—one of which he helped to create!

The Global Health Council and APHA job fairs are the places to start collecting information about consulting firms. Some even hold initial interviews at the Council's annual meeting. Most now have web sites and sophisticated marketing materials that can give you a sense of the organization's strong suits and corporate culture.

6. Local Government Agencies and Indigenous Non-Governmental Organizations (NGOs)

More and more international health professionals are finding work overseas with local non-governmental organizations (NGOs) and host country government agencies. If you're lucky enough to work with this type of organization, you'll probably be shoulder to shoulder with local leaders.

With the 1979 Alma Alta commitment to "Health for all by the Year 2000," world leaders realized that the development of sustainable primary health care programs depended on establishing and enhancing local institutions, both public and private. These are the government agencies and local NGOs that will continue when the funding and support from foreign PVOs and international donors are no longer available or necessary.

Even the poorest country has a government agency responsible for health care. However, anyone who has walked into a ministry of health in a developing country can see the challenges government health workers face. Underpaid and overextended, successful public officials have become extremely skilled at keeping programs going with minimal resources. One way involves collaborating with private nongovernmental organizations, or NGOs.

NGOs are locally-established private groups, loosely modeled on their US-based PVO cousins and just as varied in their structures, missions, services, and the people they serve. Thousands of NGOs have been established worldwide since the mid-1980s. While some floundered or died, many have survived and become key players in the health care systems within their countries.

As private organizations that often represent the interests of indigenous peoples, minorities, or others lacking access to health care, many NGOs find themselves in conflict with their government and have become strong advocates for the rights of their people.

Both the NGOs and the public sector health care systems have begun to look to the multilateral agencies (such as the UN and World Bank) and the PVOs for assistance, both financial and technical. Primary technical areas of need include organizational development, strategic planning, program evaluation, administration, and fundraising.

Here's where you can come in. Staff from the international organizations are "seconded" or loaned out to the local NGO or government agency for a period of time. They play the role of mentor, usually to senior level management. You'll be best suited for these roles if you have been working in the country for some time and have the language skills and the cultural acumen to fit in.

When Americans are hired from the US, it is usually through a third agency or organization that is working with the local entity. This is not to say that you can't establish connections with local groups on your own and offer your services. Again, making contact requires creativity. In many cultures, a letter from a stranger offering to help is viewed skeptically. The best way is to work through intermediaries or contacts working inside the agency, who know your work and the people there. Personal connections are more powerful than even the most articulate letter.

The level of salary and benefits you can expect from a government agency or an NGO largely depends on who is sitting opposite you when you sign your contract. Obviously, if you're working with the NGO or local government agency as a seconded employee from the U.N. or a PVO, you will make far more than you would working directly for the local entity.

7. US Government

If you're pretty serious about global health as a career, you'll want to explore the many employment options within the US government, including (but not limited to) the Department of State's Foreign Service, the US Agency for International Development, the National Institutes of Health, the Centers for Disease Control and Prevention, and the various branches of the US armed forces.

While an exhaustive look at all of these options is way beyond the scope of this book, in general, employment with the government at all but the lowest level will involve some testing, security clearances and dealing with a slow bureaucracy.

A good place to start to investigate the possibilities is at the website www.usajobs.opm.gov. This is the official site for employment information and jobs listed with the federal Office of Personnel Management. The best way to navigate the site is to go to "Advanced Search" and look at jobs by agency.

8. Multilateral Agencies

Multilateral (multiple countries involved) agencies like the Pan American Health Organization or the World Health Organization, for example, are the titans of global health. With billion dollar budgets, these agencies carry out programs and projects in every corner of the world, deploying thousands of staff and wielding enormous influence.

Although health program officer positions with the United Nations and the World Health Organization are highly sought-after (and often highly politicized), there are possibilities for entry level work. An excellent directory is located at http://icsc.un.org/joblinks.asp, which links you to listings of all job, volunteer and internship possibilities within the UN system. Many of these are directly involved in global health.

If you're working on a graduate degree in a relevant field, you may want to explore possible internships with the World Health Organization. These unpaid positions provide an opportunity for students to expand their understanding of WHO's goals, policies and activities.

Interns cover their own costs of medical insurance, travel and accommodation, as well as living expenses. As an intern, you are also responsible for obtaining the necessary visas and arranging travel. The time frame is 6 to 12 weeks, and you can not apply for a UN job for at least three months after completing your internship.

According to the WHO, the majority of students are placed in health-related programs, although there are very limited opportunities in general administrative areas such as translation. It helps to be in a health field. For more info, check www.who.int/employment/internship.

Stepping outside the box

If none of the above seems like the right path to you, but you're still set on a career in global health, you must be one of those truly adventurous spirits. Don't despair. Others before you have boarded a plane and gone overseas to work, without a job, contacts, or even much money. But remember, if you take this route, you've got to get your own work visa, arrange your medical evacuation insurance, and contend with myriad other details. It's not easy, but for the truly driven, it can be an option.

Some who are both adventurous and entrepreneurial have taken an even bigger leap, by starting their own humanitarian organizations. Interestingly, many who opt for this are not your typical international development professionals. They are more often people new to global humanitarian work: business executives taking early retirement, or even immigrants wanting to help out in their homeland. Read Segundo and Joan Velasquez' story after Chapter Six to see how one couple acted on their desire to help out.

This approach is not for everyone. Fundraising, getting approval from a government to run a project in their country, even filing for tax-exempt status in the US so you can raise money—can all take longer and cost more than you probably imagine. But if you've examined the organizations that are already out there and none of them seem to do exactly what you think needs doing, then go for it!

BERT HIRSCHHORN
"I went, and it turned out well"

As a medical student in the early 1960s, I had the idea that I wanted to be a medical missionary. I planned to go to Alaska. The funny thing was I was a Jewish kid, an immigrant from Austria, and I had no idea that to be a medical missionary you have to be a Christian. Which gives you an indication of how naive I was!

One of my professors at Boston Hospital was very interested in international health. This was at the beginning of the Vietnam War, and of course I got called up. For doctors, an alternative was to join the Public Health Service. Through this, the National Institutes of Health had an international research career development program. My mentor encouraged me to do hepatitis research, so I decided to go to Ghana. I had a research program all set up. I was ready to discover the viral cause of hepatitis B. If I had pursued that, I

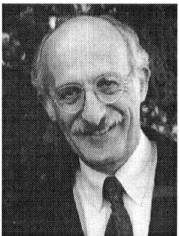

Bert helped develop Oral Rehydration Therapy, which has saved millions of lives.

could have won the Nobel Prize. (It was awarded to Dr. Baruch Blumberg.) But there was political upheaval in Ghana and they decided not to send me.

The NIH bureaucrat said to me" You'll go to Pakistan and study diarrhea, instead." I said "Diarrhea! That's the last thing I want to do!" I had spent six months preparing to go to Ghana, I had studied the different tribes, I knew about the languages. He said "You'll get a free car, free housing." That stuff didn't interest me. I was very idealistic. I didn't want to go, but I went, and it turned out well. All my life I've done well, just by backing into things.

So I went to the Cholera Research Laboratory in Pakistan. Cholera kills because the victim gets totally dehydrated, usually through incredible, massive diarrhea. This was a problem: how to rehydrate patients? Typically, they had been rehydrated intravenously, with a mixture of salt and sugar. I understood the science and physiology of this process, and being up to speed on medical science has always stood me in good stead. Researchers had just developed a better rehydration solution, but it was still being done intravenously. I read a lot of the literature about how glucose and sodium are absorbed in the gut. My colleagues and I wondered, "Can rehydration be done by mouth?"

This was not really the right time to ask this question. In fact at the time, NIH wanted to embargo any further research on oral rehydration, because US Navy researchers had tried oral rehydration a few years earlier in the Phillipines and it had been a total failure. Eight or nine patients died. Coincidentally, the head of that research project was now the director of the Cholera Research Laboratory. I wanted his permission to take another look at the study. He said, "You absolutely cannot try this again. It doesn't work!" I asked to see his results. Looking at them, I could tell that you had to give a solution orally that was like the new IV solution. He had been giving them something that was way too concentrated. I explained this, and since we were in the middle of an epidemic, and we were running out of IV fluids, he let me try oral rehydration again with just a few patients. I had to sleep in the same room with them, and we had to keep an IV line in, just in case.

It worked! We published the results in the New England Journal of Medicine in 1968. At first we didn't realize how far-reaching this discovery was. Until Oral RehydrationTherapy (ORT) was used during the Bangladesh refugee crisis, we didn't know that people who were rehydrated using ORT could do as well or better than those with intravenous lines.

▲ ▲ ▲

I returned to the U.S. realizing that although I was good at research, I really wanted a bigger stage, more interaction with people all over the world. Lab work has the potential to turn you into a real solitaire. The National Institutes of Health had been doing a lot of research with Indians on reservations. The Indians were getting the sense that was all we were interested in—research. We needed something that was more community-based. So they asked me to introduce ORT to the White Mountain Apache Nation, where the infant mortality rate was still an incredibly high 75 per 1,000.

So I took two teams of providers to Arizona over two long summers. We did lots of different work out there, clinical, environmental, training people. I loved it. We continued to explore the various uses of ORT, too, showing that it could be used to treat very young infants, and that it actually improved the nutritional status of patients.

It was on the White Mountain Reservation that I learned about the public health approach. I saw that all the public health nurses I worked with were thinking about denominators, and I was still thinking only about numerators. I realized, I can't go back to hospital work any more.

▲ ▲ ▲

I left Johns Hopkins University to join Management Sciences for Health (MSH), an international public health consulting group in Boston. It was a total risk, because consulting groups were not popular with academics. But at that point, everything began to take off. At MSH we launched a bunch of different programs: the essential drug program, among others. I got into family planning, quality of care assessment, and I wrote a couple of books on that topic.

In 1975 we were asked to help the World Health Organization design a rural clinic study in the Philippines on ORT. We started teaching people in the clinics, and the nurses spread the education to shopkeepers, and finally we were teaching mothers in their homes, who could show their neighbors how to do it. It's really that simple.

In 1978, six of us broke off from Management Sciences for Health and started our own consulting firm, called John Snow, Incorporated. We named it after the famous English epidemiologist who tracked the cause of a London cholera epidemic to a particular tainted water pump. With JSI, I went to Egypt to direct a diarrheal disease control project for the Egyptian government. It succeeded beyond expectations and its success led to other, large scale public health projects in immunization and child survival. John Snow has grown phenomenally. From six of us in 1978, it now has a staff of over 500. My founding partner, Joel Lamstein, still directs it. I'm now a sort of "emeritus" partner.

▲ ▲ ▲

In 1990 I followed my wife to her job in Indonesia with the Ford Foundation. I didn't really know what I was going to do. But soon I was asked by the Food and Agricultural Organization (FAO) to do a study on health risks to farmers who used pesticides. We showed quite clearly that the farmers, who would apply liquid pesticides by hand, were being acutely poisoned. What's more, they knew it. It wasn't a matter of "health education." They knew they were handling poisons, but they couldn't afford protective clothing. Even if they could have afforded it, you can't wear a full suit of protective gear, face mask and boots, in a tropical rice paddy. We showed that they were being poisoned by economic necessity, the cost of doing business. This led to some important reforms: last year the FAO finalized an international convention saying that companies can not export pesticides to other countries that are banned in their country of origin. Again, a good "accident" led to some good work.

▲ ▲ ▲

After three years, I came to Minnesota, of all places, because that's where my wife has family, and because I was invited by the University of Minnesota to teach a course in international public health as a visiting professor. After my contract ended there, I joined the Minnesota Department of Health. I was asked to energize the division of family health, and I think we succeeded. I worked with some really dedicated people. I learned about a whole range of public health I'd not explored before: alcohol abuse, tobacco control, cardiovascular disease, diabetes *prevention and more. It was like getting an MPH. Better, even. It's true that until you've been a public health bureaucrat, you don't know what public health is all about. Unfortunately, I also learned that in a more painful way, when I tried to protect my staff from a governor's wife who had decided she knew better than we did about a particular topic. I was ordered off my position and offered another post, but I knew it was a charade, so I refused, and let myself be fired.*

It was a principled stand, but it wasn't easy. I was 60 years old, not sure what I would do next. I still had work left in me. It was a hard period. But then my wife went off to work in Geneva for a few months, and the World Health Organization offered me some consulting work, anaylzing tobacco industry documents uncovered by Minnesota's tobacco trials. I was really documenting what multinational tobacco corporations have planned for marketing cigarettes in developing countries. These papers are very revealing. It's really incredible how amoral these companies are. I call it "George Orwell meets Josef Goebbels."

▲ ▲ ▲

People sometimes say to me, "How do you do all this stuff? It must be that you're incredibly smart." Honestly, I don't think it's about being smart. I don't think I'm smarter than many other people. But I am an enormous autodidact. I always want to figure out a new way of doing something. To do this work, you have to be teaching yourself all the time. You have to be a leech, to stick on to people who are willing to mentor you. And you have to record what you've done. Without a record, no one can learn from it. Being open to new experiences, backing into things, reading, writing, learning. That isn't just what it takes to succeed in international public health—that's what it takes to be an intelligent person, which, it seems to me, is the highest human capacity.

Editor's note: Since this interview, Bert has made his home in Beirut and Helsinki, while teaching global health courses at Yale University. He writes poetry and continues his research on the global marketing of tobacco products.

CHAPTER SIX

Landing That First Assignment

You've made up your mind: you really want to go. You know which types of organizations interest you, and you've begun to broaden your network. Maybe you've started to test the waters, using the tips in Chapter Four. So, what's next? Finding the right job for yourself!

In this chapter, you will learn how to land that first assignment. You'll read how to:
- find the organization that's right for you;
- tailor your resume, cover letters and interviews to highlight what global health employers are looking for;
- ace job interviews, both on the phone and in person; and
- ask the crucial questions before you sign any employment contract or volunteer agreement.

Start now!

First, though, we'll clue you in about a few things you should start doing immediately—or as soon as you are almost 100% sure that you'll be leaving town within six months. Once you've decided that you want to work overseas, you should make these preparations, even if you don't yet have a position. Global health employers are often in a rush to get someone into the field ASAP. Having these details taken care of now can smooth the process later.

1. Check your passport.

Make sure you have a passport that has an expiration date at least twelve months past the date you hope to go overseas. Some countries will not issue you an entry visa if your passport is near expiration. Also, make copies of the title page and visas, when you get them. When you pack up, hide copies in several places throughout your luggage. Having a copy can make it much easier to get replacement passports and visas, should you lose them.

2. Start getting your shots now.

Some of the vaccines you will need require up to six months to complete. Make an appointment with your local travel or international clinic—make sure it's a place with links to the Centers for Disease Control, for up-to-date health advisories.

Tell your provider you are contemplating work in a developing country in the near future and that you are interested in getting the appropriate vaccines. If you can at least pinpoint a region, so much the better.

Ask for a yellow World Health Organization International

Certificate of Vaccination card, which you will want to take with you. Many countries require this particular card as proof that you are immunized.

3. Get some mug shots, too.
It's always a good idea to have a few current passport-sized photos handy when traveling. These are necessary when applying for visas and other documents in-country. Take them now, and you'll have time to get them taken again when they inevitably come back looking awful.

> **START NOW!**
> *1. Check your passport.*
> *2. Start getting your shots.*
> *3. Get some mug shots, too.*
> *4. Look official.*
> *5. Learn four on the floor.*
> *6. Get your affairs in order.*
> *7. Consult your accountant.*

4. Look official.
Many countries require foreign doctors, nurses and other licensed health professionals to present originals of their diplomas, licenses and certificates for review before they are allowed to practice. Rather than risk losing these precious documents, consider making some good copies and sprucing them up with ribbons or a special embossing stamp, so they look like the original.

5. Learn four on the floor.
Knowing how to drive a stick shift (maybe one that's missing a few gears) should be a standard requirement of all global health training programs. If you only drive an automatic, start learning now how to grind those gears. Also, go to your local AAA office to get an International Drivers Permit. This can help if you get into trouble driving overseas, although you still may need a local license.

6. Get your affairs in order.

Find someone you can trust with your possessions and personal finances. Do you have a will, a living will, disability insurance? Should you rent a safety deposit box for your valuables?

7. Consult your accountant.

Find out about the tax and financial ramifications of going overseas, either as an employee or as a volunteer. If you have student loans, are you still liable for them, or can they be deferred?

Which place is right for you?

Now you can begin in earnest to identify which organizations seem like the best fit for you, and once you've done that, to strengthen your application. The short version is: learn everything you can about the organizations that sound right. The more you know about the history, mission, and challenges of an organization, the more effective you can make your appeal for a job and the less likely you are to have a nasty surprise later on.

Take these three steps to become a more informed creator of your global health future:

1. Join the Global Health Council

The Global Health Council is the world's largest membership alliance dedicated to improving health throughout the world. Its diverse membership includes individuals (health care professionals and students) and organizations (NGOs, foundations, government agencies and academic institutions.) Visit their website, www.globalhealth.org, to find out what the Council does and how you can get involved.

The Council offers valuable resources for job seekers:

The organization's website has a *Career Network* where you can learn about current jobs and internships. You can also submit your own resume to be viewed by recruiters.

The Council's annual conference in Washington DC, traditionally held the first week in June, provides a great opportunity to network with practitioners and the leading organizations involved in global health. Special sessions are held during the conference for those interested in a career. The price of registration can be steep but there are student and retiree rates, and a discount for folks who volunteer to help out at the conference site. If you are ready to get serious about a job search, attending the conference will be worth your time and money. Go to www.globalhealth.org/conference to sign up.

Two Council publications, *The Global Health Directory* and the *Global AIDS Directory*, include listings of organizations that offer internship and volunteer opportunities for those exploring the field of global health. Both publications are described and can be ordered on the Council's website.

2. Get on the Internet.

The Internet has dramatically changed the field of global health in just the past five years. Nearly every organization involved in this field and even many of their projects now have their own websites, with information, stories and photos. Many offer a means to communicate one-on-one with staff. Increasingly, such organizations use their websites as a primary recruitment and screening tool for potential hires. (Read more on this in the next section, Getting Your Foot in the Door.)

Given all that, there really is no excuse for not knowing about the organizations you are applying to. Do your research before making that first contact!

Don't be daunted by the public relations threaded throughout many of these sites; it's reasonable for organizations to want to play up their strengths. Comparing promotional approaches among organizations can be revealing, helping you to understand the mission, work sites, philosophy of development, programs, funding sources, and approach to raising money of each agency that appeals to you.

3. Interview former volunteers and staff.

Every organization has its own culture, which you can best understand from the perspective of someone who's worked there. The information you'll find on an organization's website and in their printed materials is the public face. Former volunteers and staff can often give you a more personal view.

Where can you find these wellsprings of information? They're everywhere, attending conferences, teaching in universities, speaking at local churches, working at public health departments or clinics, typing away in chat rooms, volunteering with local organizations—maybe even taking out your appendix! You can start to build your network by contacting the agency you're interested in, and asking if any former staffers live in your area. Especially with larger organizations, like Peace Corps, you're apt to find someone nearby.

When you do find an alumnus of an organization that you're interested in, schedule time for a coffee break (you pay). Most people enjoy telling about their experiences overseas. You shouldn't have much trouble getting the conversation going. Here is a list of questions to consider. If they seem useful, you may want to copy this list and bring it along.

Start with some questions about the organization, such as:
- Why did you choose the organization?
- What was the organization's work history in your country of interest?
- What was the organization's reputation and relationship with the people they were serving?
- How did the organization deal with difficulties in-country, or unexpected problems?
- Would you work with this organization again?
- What was the organization's structure? What was it like working with the director, board members, other staff?
- Which staffers were the most interesting to work with? Are they still with the organization?
- What was the most difficult aspect of working with this organization?
- Did the organization have any hidden agendas?
- Was the organization financially viable?
- Did the organization do what they said they would do in your contract, and on the project?
- Who should I be talking to first in the organization if I want to work there?
- What was the relationship between the home office and the field program?
- How flexible and supportive was the home office in helping you prepare to go overseas and then return?
- Are you still in contact with anyone from the organization?

You'll also want to ask about the alum's program focus, whether it was child survival, policy consultation, refugee relief or something else.

- Where did you work and what did you do?
- What difficulties did the program face?
- Was the program evaluated? What were its strengths and weaknesses?
- Did the program change as a result of the evaluation?
- Who funds the program? What role do they have in it?
- Is the program still running? If not, how did it end? If so, what plans are there for the future?
- What were the dynamics between the local and international staff?
- Were you replaced when you left? If so, by whom— a local or another expatriate?

And finally, you'll want the lowdown on how your interviewee fared personally:
- How did you get the job?
- What was a typical day like?
- Did you have any security concerns?
- Did you get sick? What kind of health care did you have for yourself and your family?
- Was the pay you received enough to live on?
- What expenses were covered by the organization (health insurance, vacation, sick leave)?
- Was there a grievance policy if you had problems with other staff or volunteers?
- What kinds of material things did you wish you had brought with you?
- How much free time did you have, and what did you do during your free time? (Is there access to movies, internet, books, beaches, etc.)
- Do you have any advice for someone contemplating overseas work?

Remember, every informational interview should conclude with a sincere thank you (especially if you ask all of the questions above!) and a request for more names and contact numbers of people you can talk to. A written thank-you note or email is an excellent follow-up. And if the interview has gone pleasantly, it doesn't hurt to ask if your informant knows of any interesting job openings.

Getting your foot in the door

Once you've got a list of prospective organizations developed from the Global Health Council listings, the internet and your interviews, it's time to contact them. This can be a challenge. The hard reality is that many health organizations are flooded with would-be employees, receiving anywhere from 100 to 200 unsolicited resumes a month, and over 100 responses to postings for entry level positions.

You'll have to be resourceful and creative to make your application stand out. Here are some initial steps you can take to make sure your inquiry doesn't get shelved:

1. Learn about the organizations.

Learn everything you can about the organizations you are interested in, including their mission, history, programs and what they are looking for in employees and volunteers. At this stage, this is best done by visiting websites.

2. Get on the mailing list and list servs.

Contact the organizations that sound the most interesting and ask to be added to their mailing lists (postal and e-mail) and list servs. This is an excellent way to keep up to speed on new programs and possible job openings.

3. Give a little.

Make a donation in cash or spend some time in the home

FOR GREAT RESUMES
1. Tailor your resume to the job.
2. Explain your acronynms.
3. Go long, not short.
4. Highlight your travels.
5. Be accurate about languages.
6. Focus on their needs.
7. Mention your references.
8. Brag about your contacts.
9. Talk about the organization.
10. Highlight your soft side.
11. Be a storyteller.
12. Electrify your resume.
13. Proofread it all.

office. Being able to say that you're a contributor or past volunteer can help make your application stand out among all the others.

Applications that capture attention

The next step is to prepare your resume. Because of the growing number of positions and applicants, more organizations are computerizing their recruitment processes. Many places have a database where you enter your information online. This allows the organization to process, store and retrieve many more applications. Other organizations continue to accept hard copies of resumes. Regardless of the method used to convey your experience, it's best to start by updating your resume. Here are some tips:

1. Tailor your resume to the position.

Most recruiters work from a checklist of absolute job requirements and preferred qualifications. If you are responding to a posting that requires French, be sure to mention your level of fluency (and don't apply unless you are truly fluent!). Be understanding of the recruiter (who may be reading 50 resumes a day) by clearly responding to all the job requirements in both your cover letter and resume.

2. *Explain the acronyms you use.*
Don't assume that the person reading your materials will know the jargon. Refer to the World Health Organization in full before abbreviating it as WHO, for example.

3. *Go longer, rather than short.*
A two to four page resume is fine. In international work, it is not uncommon for people to change organizations and assignments every two to four years. This can lengthen a resume, especially for someone in the 15th or 20th year of their career. If your resume is long, add a brief summary at the beginning, responding to the requirements of the specific job.

4. *Highlight your world travels.*
List all of the countries where you've worked, even for relatively short assignments of one month or less.

5. *Be accurate about your language skills.*
If you speak multiple languages, list them all, including English. Highlight those in which you are fluent.

6. *Focus on their needs, not yours.*
Omit special needs (i.e. special health care, schools, etc.) at this point. These issues are better left to the interview.

7. *Mention your references.*
Include a list of references with the resume. It can save time in the long run. Make sure the names and contact information are current and if possible, that at least one of your references can be reached easily in the US. Explain how and when overseas contacts can be reached. Include e-mail addresses as well as phone numbers whenever possible.

8. Brag about your contacts—selectively.

Connections are key. Slipping the names of people you know who have worked with the organization into your cover letter and reference list may help keep your resume in the pile and out of the can. Be sure that the people you mention are well-regarded, however!

9. Talk about the organization.

Demonstrating in your cover letter that you know the organization and their needs will help, too. This is where thorough research can really pay off, and a generic letter will fail. Of course, it never hurts to have demonstrated interest as a donor to an organization.

10. Highlight your soft side.

Stress—with relevant examples—the "soft skills" organizations are always looking for, including flexibility, self direction, consistency with the organization's values, ability to work in stressful situations, cross-cultural work experience, and optimism.

11. Be a storyteller.

Don't lie—but be creative about your experiences. Illustrative stories or situations can be helpful and can often make the cover letter more memorable.

12. Electrify your resume.

More and more organizations prefer electronic versus hard copy resumes, since the former are easier to file and retrieve.

13. Proofread before you send.

With word processing programs that cut and paste, you can now send your resume to nearly every employer on the planet with a click of a button. Make sure you send your application to only one organizaation per email, and check the address before you send.

Why don't they return all my calls?

If you're calling an organization repeatedly in the hope that persistence will pay off, *stop.* This approach will seldom work in the global health field. Let's face it, you may never get a response, especially with an unsolicited resume, but even if you are responding to a posted position.

It's a buyer's market. But don't let that stop you from writing to the organization with updated information as your situation (your address, experience, etc) changes. If you live elsewhere, it's fair to call an agency when you're in town, to set up an informational interview.

First interviews

They've got your resume and you've just received a call to set up an interview. Terrific! You've survived the first major hurtle. But you don't have that job yet, and your interview can make or break it. Here are some pointers:

1. Take your time.

Usually, the first interview is done over the phone. If you are called for an interview, don't get too excited and start the interview right away. Reschedule it. That'll give you the time necessary to get focused, organize your points, and recall what you said in your cover letter.

2. Showcase your second language.

If a second language is required, expect to conduct at least a part of the interview in that language. If your interviewer doesn't ask, suggest it.

UNFORGETTABLE INTERVIEWS
1. Take your time.
2. Showcase your second language.
3. Be clear about your motives.
4. Tell a good story.
5. Translate theory into practice.
6. Stress your writing skills.
7. Be curious.
8. Know your timeline.
9. Finally, get personal.

3. Be clear about your motives.

Be prepared to explain in a compelling way why you want to work overseas. (Remember your motivations from Chapter Three!)

4. Tell a good story.

As with your cover letter, prepare an anecdote or two that is based on your past experience: one that relates to the position requirements and shows you in a favorable light. At the end of a long day, when the recruiter has interviewed a dozen similarly qualified candidates over the phone, a memorable story can make you stand out.

5. Translate theory into practice.

Some organizations use case studies in their interviews to describe specific challenges and ask you how you would respond. Again, being able to relate a story about a relevant past experience is far more memorable and entertaining than a "textbook" answer. If you don't have an experience to offer, be creative and take your time in responding. Feel free to ask questions about the situation and add to the story to make it unique.

6. Stress your writing skills.

Offer copies of your writing, both in English and in any required second language.

7. *Be curious.*

At some point in the interview, politely turn the tables, and ask some questions of your interviewers. This shows an understanding of how programs operate and demonstrates your interest in the organization and the position.

8. *Know your timeline.*

Be ready to discuss possible departure and return dates. Make sure you have time for work, housing, and business arrangements, and to set up your children's schooling.

9. *Finally, get personal.*

The best time to mention any special needs (disability, special education for children, major family problems) is toward the end of the first interview when you sense things are going well.

Second interviews

If the organization wants you to come to the home office for a second, face-to-face interview, a big question usually is who pays for the trip. Decide beforehand if you are willing to cover the costs of a trip to the home office. If the organization pays, you're almost guaranteed the red eye special— round trip to and from, on the same day.

Be prepared for a long day! Face to face interviews at the home office can be grueling— early or late flights, taxi cabs, hotel rooms, and all day in meetings, being shuttled from person to person and from department to department. Be especially courteous to secretaries and assistants who may be shepherding you around. Sure, it's good karma, but it's also good strategy.

Try to remain flexible and charming, no matter how exhausted you get. The decision rests now more on the personal dynamics between you and the people in the organization. The bottom line at this point is whether they feel they can trust you enough to send you half way around the world, and whether you can trust them to provide the necessary support. And the fact is, a grueling day of interviews may be a walk in the park compared to some of the days you'll have in the field. Get used to it.

Your interviewers will ask a lot about you, but now's your chance to ask some important questions of your own. Be sure to cover the questions below to your satisfaction. They may seem redundant, but the answers may confirm or deny what you've already learned through research and interviews.

First, hone in on the project you're being considered for:
- What are the goals of the project?
- What are its major challenges?
- Is this project time limited?
- Are there plans for turning it over to local nationals?
- Where does the organization get its funding?
- How is this project being funded?
- Are national staff involved, and how?
- Has there been a lot of turnover in the past?
- How secure is the funding?

Then ask specifically about the job.
- What, exactly, are the job duties?
- Is this a new position or am I replacing someone else?
- If a replacement, why are they leaving and can there be an overlap period?
- Who will I report to and supervise?
- Will I be working with a local counterpart?

- How is this position funded and for how long?
- Will I be expected to raise money?
- Why isn't this position going to a national?
- What is the security situation?

Don't take someone else's job.

In many developing countries, the number of trained doctors, nurses, and public health professionals has grown dramatically over the past 20 years. Yet sadly, many remain unemployed or under-employed, even as international organizations send workers overseas.

The decision to send an American—as opposed to hiring a local professional— should be raised during your interview. In many global health projects, the international volunteer or employee is paired up with a local counterpart, where the latter can learn specific skills to use when the international leaves.

Lastly, ask the tough questions:
- What is the pay and what expenses are covered?
- What are the living arrangements?
- What about time off and vacation time?
- How will I communicate with the home office, as well as family and friends in the US?
- Can my contract be extended?
- What if I need to come home unexpectedly?
- When and how will contract decisions be made?

Signing up

The interviews have gone swimmingly, and the organization is offering you a job or a volunteer position. Congratulations! But before you pack your expedition gear, look closely at your contract or volunteer agreement. Don't sign a thing until you are clear on the following:

- Who covers and makes the travel arrangements? Who pays for immunizations and other medical expenses? Are medical evacuation insurance and health insurance provided?

- How and where will you be paid? In local currency or US dollars? What kind of banking facilities are available? If payments are in local currency, what arrangements can be made to protect the value of your salary against currency devaluations?

- What other costs are covered? Taxes, transport to and from for yourself, your family, and your personal things; in-country travel on busines; use of project vehicles for personal transport; living allowance, paid vacation and home leave? (Some organizations are able to get student loan deferrments for their volunteers. Check the financial affairs office at your school and the agency that's offering to hire you.)

As in any employment situation, don't leap from your current position until you get a signed contract or offer.

JOAN and SEGUNDO VELAZQUEZ
"No one did what we wanted to do"

Segundo: I'm from Bolivia, from Cochabamba, which is way up in the Andes. I came to the United States and ended up working for Northwest Airlines. Working for the airline provided me the opportunity to travel at little cost to Bolivia, so I often visited my family there. And I was always struck by the great need there and the great surplus here. Eighty percent of the people there live below subsistence level. In some rural areas, up to a third of the children die before the age of five.

My brother is a doctor, and so one day we started talking about how we might be able to help him and others who provide care to the poor. I started by carrying down some medical instruments, just a few things that I could carry in my pockets, practically. The next time, six months later, I carried stuff in an extra carry-on bag. Then it was a suitcase, then two packing boxes, then 28 boxes. Then we called in the National Guard! Seriously, when we started we had no idea we would grow so quickly, and that we would be handling so many supplies.

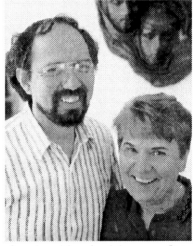

Segundo and Joan founded a non-profit to collect supplies for re-use in Bolivia.

Joan: Our organization grew equally informally. It started with just Segundo and me and a few friends and family members in the US and Bolivia. Then we discovered that a great deal more surplus material could be recycled to Bolivia through a formal organization. We contacted other organizations working in Bolivia, thinking that they might be able to channel our supplies to clinics and hospitals. But they all had their own programs and specific ways of operating. So finally, when we realized that no organization existed to do what we wanted to do, we formed a non-profit organization, Mano a Mano (Hand to Hand Medical Resources).

Segundo: *We exist to bring medical equipment and supplies to Bolivians who need them. We collect and recyle material that would otherwise be discarded in the US. All kinds of things: beds, sheets, gowns, walkers, syringes, gloves, bandages, x-ray machines, gurneys. Anything you can imagine using in a hospital or clinic, except medications.*

In the beginning, the Bolivian NGO in which my brother Jose was working was able to distribute 90 percent of what we sent down. During the first three years, we completely upgraded a 32 bed hospital, an outpatient clinic that sees 33,000 patients yearly, and five satellite clinics operated by that NGO in Cochabamba! This was already far beyond what we thought we could do.

Joan: *When we started, I spent a whole summer reading IRS regulations and the rules for the creation of a non-profit. We organized a board of directors and incorporated. Our biggest break came when we learned about the Denton Program, a USAID supported program that allows military transport planes to ship humanitarian goods at no cost. That meant we could get medical inventory into Bolivia with minimal transportation costs.*

The most complicated aspect of our work has been dealing with the bureaucracy related to customs. As complicated as it is dealing with regulations on the US side, it was even more so on the Bolivian end, where regulations change constantly, and where your dealings are all based on personal relationships.

Segundo: *Health care facilities in the US are paying to get rid of stuff that we can use. One hospital we called had incinerated 70 mattresses, the day before we called them. What constitutes a solid waste problem for them is actually desperately needed medical equipment in Bolivia. Americans get a new set of crutches every time they sprain an ankle. Goodwill donates to us all their discarded sets of crutches, to send them down to Bolivia.*

Once we understood how to go about collecting the surplus, it was incredible how much there was. In our first months of operation we had wondered whether we would be able to get 2,000 pounds to ship, which is the minimum under the Denton Program. Our last shipment a few months ago was 90,000 pounds!

Joan: We work out of our home, with the help of about 90 volunteers. No one is paid anything here in the US, although we do have two part-time employees at the warehouse in Bolivia. We bought a forklift last year to help move the pallets around here in the US. Right now we've got over 400 boxes of supplies and many pallets of equipment in our garage and basement, waiting for the next shipment. Every Friday we sort things that we have picked up during the week. It's like Christmas once a week. You never know what you're going to unpack. Yesterday we got a shipment of the most beautiful occupational therapy boards. No one in Bolivia has even seen anything like them.

Segundo: Since 1997, we've helped to build five clinics. The first one was not part of our work plan: One of our Board members wanted to do something to honor a volunteer on her 70th birthday. We had a party and suggested that contributions be made to Mano a Mano in her name, to construct a clinic. We collected enough to provide seed funding for the construction of two clinics to be located in desperately poor communities surrounding Cochabamba.

Joan: Our idea is that eventually either a Bolivian NGO or the community itself will take over the management of the clinics. That has happened with two of them already. We want to stay small; we don't want to outstrip the capacity of our US volunteers or our Bolivian counterparts. But we'd like to think about other kinds of community development, maybe to start a greenhouse project, or a micro-loan project, to increase the self-sufficiency of the people using the clinics.

Segundo: It's been very rewarding. So many people don't want all of these wonderful things to go to waste. It's been satisfying to see the impact it can have in Bolivia. Because we have family and friends involved, we know we are cost-effective, too. Things are not being pilfered and they are not ending up on the black market.

Joan: *It's an enormous amount of work. I spend 40 hours a week on Mano a Mano, and Segundo probably puts in 20 hours a week. But it's worth it. The biggest personal reward came one day when I saw photos of an entire clinic that had been furnished with supplies and equipment from Mano a Mano. It is so gratifying to see the stuff that we pick up and pack and load into boxes, being used, everything even down to the curtains!*

Editor's note: As of early 2005, Mano a Mano had built 45 primary care clinics in rural Bolivia, with continued major funding from an anonymous donor. In 2004, the organization's first full-time US employee was hired. Joan and Segundo continue to work full-time as volunteer co-directors. To find out more about Mano a Mano Medical Resources, visit the website, www.manoamano.org.

CHAPTER SEVEN

Getting Ready To Go

Congratulations, you're hired! Time to get packing. What needs to happen before you leave? What do you bring? What do you leave behind? Who do you tell? Who'll take care of the dog? Should you sell the house or turn it over to relatives? The list of decisions can seem endless as your departure date approaches.

In this chapter, we'll help you prepare for going overseas, covering the following topics:
- learning more about your destination;
- organizing the last minute chores and deciding what to bring;
- preparing yourself physically and mentally; and
- special considerations when taking children along.

Where did you say you were headed?

Learning about your destination can be one of the most enjoyable and invigorating aspects of preparation. It can also be a great way to share the experience with your family and friends, whether or not they're going with you. There are a variety of resources to investigate for information and inspiration. Below, some suggestions:

Travel guidebooks and maps

They exist for almost every country or region on the globe. Although targeted primarily to tourists, they can also be a helpful resource for professionals going overseas to work or volunteer. One of the most popular series is the *Lonely Planet* guides (www.lonelyplanet.com). These are excellent on practical information about culture, history, geography, and sightseeing junkets. Their bibliographies are also good for further reading.

One of the shortfalls of any travel guidebook is the accuracy and timeliness of the information. Things change, often overnight. New governments come into power, the security situation heats up, the exchange rate drops through the floor, cutting your paycheck in half. All this and more can happen between the editions of guidebooks. So, verify, verify, verify.

Universities

Colleges and universities can often connect you with foreign students or faculty from the area where you're planning to work. International clubs, libraries and travel/study centers may provide additional helpful contacts.

Language Programs

The more you can learn of the local language, the better. Clarify early on whether the organization sending you will cover language study. Even if you are terrible with languages, the effort you put in will be appreciated and can only broaden your understanding of the culture. If you've got the time and the money, language immersion programs are an excellent way to develop basic language skills. Other options include tutors (maybe you can swap tutoring with a foreign student at your local college) and language tapes.

Internet

Newspapers from all over the world are establishing their own websites. The quality and content are inconsistent, usually focusing on the extremes, from the mundane to the gratuitous. But hey, that sounds like many of our newspapers in the US, too. If you can get a local or national newspaper from the area where you're headed, you can practice reading in the language as well.

The internet is also home to a rapidly growing array of websites and chat rooms with information on every country of the world. As with all information found on the internet, a good dose of skepticism is warranted.

The arts

Even the world's poorest countries have their own traditions in music, literature, cinema, painting, dance, sculpture, and the other fine and folk arts. Trips to your local library, book store, art museum, and video rental store can be an excellent first step for you and your family. If you have children, look for age-appropriate books, movies, and websites that you can share with them, so they can start to build their own expectations and goals for the coming trip.

Immigrant communities

There are people in your own neighborhood or town who might be a resource for you. New Americans can give you a first hand perspective on what your experience of living and working in their home country will be like.

Your new employer

The organization sending you overseas should be able to link you up to information, including staff or volunteers who have lived there, an orientation manual, and written reports. They should also help you get in contact with the field staff, who can be an excellent resource. As you work through this process, thousands of questions will come to mind. To avoid being a pest to the organization sending you, keep a notebook handy to note these questions. This can help you limit your anxious phone calls.

Last minute details

Most of us dread the final stages of trip preparation. We wait until the last minute, when the fear of forgetting something outweighs the inertia of denial and delay. Like most other things in life, the sooner you start swimming, the less your chances of sinking. Here are some thoughts on how to get started:

1. Take care of the basics.

Review the list at the beginning of Chapter Six to make sure all of those issues are being taken care of.

2. Get your visas.

Is the organization sending you overseas handling this? If not, do you know what kind of visa you need: tourist or work? Is it good for a single entry or multiple visits? This process can take time, and once you've mailed off your passport, there's little you can do to speed things along. So start early. If you don't have much time, use one of the many visa services listed on the internet, which can expedite the process, for a fee.

3. Understand your tax responsibilities.

Make sure you know what you need to do to meet tax obligations and deadlines while overseas. Inform those who need to know, including your accountant and whomever you've found to take care of your business issues while away.

4. Set up your financial system.

The organization sending you should address crucial questions about how you will handle money, such as:

- What kinds of money can be used where you'll be living? (US currency, credit cards, travelers checks, large denominations of local currency?)
- How is money exchanged and where: in banks, on the street? Is there a charge to exchange money?
- What is the current exchange rate and how much has it changed during the last year?
- Do you need to set up your own bank account incountry?
- When will your first paycheck or stipend come through?
- Will you be paid in US dollars, local currency or both?
- Will checks go to your US bank account or will you be paid in-country?

5. Establish contact points.

Find out how people can communicate with you while you're overseas. Get the name, phone number and e-mail address of the person in the organization's home office who can reach you in an emergency. Pass this information on to your family, friends, and those responsible for your business affairs.

You should also find out about possible shipping and mailing restrictions. How long does surface mail take to arrive? How should packages be sent? Are they likely to be opened en route?

6. Smooth your arrival.

Ask the home office what you're supposed to do upon arrival in-country. Will there be someone at the airport to pick you up? Do you need a formal letter of introduction from the organization for going through customs? Call the country's embassy in the US if you have questions about what you can bring in.

7. Prepare to zip through customs.

Get a separate customs letter from the organization detailing any donated medical equipment, supplies or medicines that you might be bringing with you. Make an inventory list for each piece of luggage or packing box that includes description and quantity. For medicines, it should also include expiration dates. (Do not expect people to accept donated medicines that have passed their expiration dates.)

8. Record your possessions.

Make copies of receipts for high-cost items you're taking overseas (cameras, laptop computers, expensive jewelry, etc.) to avoid having to pay import taxes upon your return. As for the stuff you're *not* taking along, (hopefully a much larger batch of possessions) you may want to make an inventory as well. Especially if you are putting items in storage, it may give you peace of mind to know what you've got packed away.

9. Check with the friendly skies.

Call the airlines you'll be using to find out luggage size,

weight, and quantity restrictions for both carry on and checked in luggage. Each company has its own rules, which can be complicated. The costs of going over the limits can be high. When an airline hits you up for the fee while you're waiting for your next flight, the options tend to be limited and painful. Getting this straight before arriving at the airport can save time, hassle and cost. Be sure to ask about special or fragile items like bikes, guitars or computers.

10. Keep an ongoing packing list.

You can use it later as your inventory list of what you're bringing. It's a good idea to run your list by the people in the field or others who have been there recently, if possible, to find out what's available locally. See our resource lists at the back of the book for ideas on what to bring along. Many consumer goods can be extremely expensive overseas, but depending on where you're going, you may be pleasantly surprised.

This is also a good opportunity to offer to bring mail and other things for the staff who are already there.

Personal preparation: the body

Taking the time to care for your own health is crucial to a positive experience overseas, whether it's for a two week trip or a life-long sojourn. As health care providers, many of us have not followed this simple advice. We're more used to working 20 hours a day and exposing ourselves to all kinds of infectious agents, so *other* people can have normal, healthy lives. This is especially true in the field of global health, where the boundaries between work and private lives are often blurred.

So, whatever your lifestyle Stateside, resolve to take care of yourself while you're overseas. Here's how to start:

1. Get your shots.

Complete your immunizations and begin taking preventive medicines as suggested by the Centers for Disease Control and Prevention. Because a full course of vaccines can take up to six months to complete, it is best to start getting your shots almost as soon as you decide to work overseas. You can learn more about the health issues you'll be facing at the CDC's website: www.cdc.gov/travel.

> **PERSONAL PREPARATION:**
> **BODY AND MIND**
> *1. Get your shots.*
> *2. Get a check-up.*
> *3. Bring a first aid kit.*
> *4. Plan for your health care.*
> *5. Check out medivac insurance.*
> *6. Plan down time after arrival.*
> *7. Anticipate homesickness.*
> *8. Start out optimistic.*
> *9. Brace yourself!*

2. Get a check-up.

Get a full physical and dental checkup well before you leave. Take care of all pending health issues. You don't want to have a tooth pulled in the back country. Get that cavity filled! Check your eyesight, if it's been giving you trouble lately. Get an extra pair of eyeglasses or contacts made, and maybe splurge on prescription sunglasses.

3. Prepare a first aid kit.

There's a checklist for a medical supply kit included in the generic packing list at the end of this book.

4. Plan for your health care.

Ask the staff overseas about access to health care where you'll be working, especially if you're bringing your children or have any chronic conditions that might require attention. Can they suggest a local physician and dentist? Will you have access to a pharmacy that can fill your prescriptions and restock your medical supply kit?

If you'll need to be responsible for your own first aid, get a copy of *Where There Is No Doctor,* an excellent book by Dr. David Werner (Hesperian Foundation, Berkeley, California.) Think too, about how you'll keep yourself healthy, and how you can recreate your usual exercise routine

5. Make sure you've got medivac insurance.

Insurance that covers the cost of transport back to the nearest moern, equipped healthcare facility is a must, especially if you are going to a remote area. Such insurance will help you get catastrophic medical care if you need it. If the worst happens, it will help your family with the costs and logistics of getting you home. Let family members who are staying behind know about how the insurance works, just in case.

6. Plan for some down time after your arrival.

Taking the time to get used to your new surroundings is time well spent. Recovering from jet lag and time changes, introducing your gut to the local parasites, and just trying to make sense of the culture, can put you into sensory overload. Allow a few days after your arrival to adjust.

Personal preparation: the mind

Although everyone's experience in working overseas is different, here are some tips on feelings you may encounter:

1. Deal with homesickness in advance.

No matter how much you fall in love with a new place, a certain amount of homesickness and loneliness is to be expected. E-mail communication with home and the constantly expanding availability of American consumer goods —junk food especially—can help provide a respite. Bringing a good stock of books, spices and seasonings, some photos and your favorite music, along with access to your hometown paper on the internet can also help ease the transition to life in a new culture.

2. Start out optimistic, so you can stay that way.

International health, as with all international humanitarian work, has been a mixed bag, with good intentions not always leading to the intended results. Things break down; programs don't go as planned; change takes a long time; and tragically, people continue to suffer and die from treatable diseases and other maladies at a horrifying rate. Continuing to seek new solutions, without giving up in the face of past shortfalls, is one of the great challenges you'll face.

3. Brace yourself!

Recognize that you are now on the verge of an incredible experience, one that is going to change you in ways that you can not imagine.

Preparing the kids

Obviously, the needs of your children have been on your mind since the beginning of this quest. Are they going or are they staying behind? Either way, their needs must be considered.

If your kids are not coming along

Begin telling them about the trip as soon as possible, whether they are going or not. If they're not going, prepare a letter to them, should anything happen to you. If you can afford it, plan now to have them come and visit you at the end of your time, or to travel back with you. Plan to write them often. Internet is great if you have access. Tell them how often they can expect to hear from you, but warn them that the mail system is sometimes unreliable. It's always great to get a stamp-covered postcard from overseas.

If your kids are coming along

The two main concerns that parents face in taking their children overseas are access to health care and schools. Where should the family live? Will you be home schooling, sending them to boarding school or enrolling the kids in local or expatriate schools? How extensive are the local health care options if you have a child with special needs? These are all questions beyond the scope of this book. Check with other staff at your sending organization to see what they recommend. A good reference work for parents taking kids along on shorter trips is *Travel With Children* (Lonely Planet Publications).

Bon voyage!

So, you're all set, or at least as set as you can be. The plane's taking off or the bus is leaving the station. Your adventure is only beginning. But before you take off, be sure to read about preparing for your return, in Chapter Eight.

HUY PHAM
"I've seen the terror and the joy of global work"

My interest in global health stems from being born in Vietnam and coming to the US at 13, with my family as refugees from the Vietnam War. This was my very first cross-cultural experience, with the immersion, getting used to the new language, and the ways of society.

As a child in Vietnam, I always got the impression that America was made up just of white people and black people. I didn't see much different than that going to high school in the suburbs (although I was certainly a novelty). But once I went to college, I met people from all races, from around the world. Some of my best friends were foreign students. My interest in overseas work started there. On campus I participated in various movements of the time—University divestment from South Africa, protesting the bombing of Libya. We formed a group that met weekly to discuss world events over beers.

Finally a friend of mine who was a former Peace Corps worker said "Huy, it's time for you to leave America again." I signed up and got sent to Liberia, in West Africa, where I worked with the rural fisheries extension service. I was supposed to be demonstrating to farmers how to raise fish in hand-dug ponds, both as a source of income and to supply extra protein for their families. The work was a lot slower than I initially expected. When I arrived, I planned that within two years a farmer I was working with would have dug six ponds; in reality, by the time I left, he was just starting to work on the third pond. There was a long acculturation phase. I couldn't really expect people to accept me after I just arrived. What did I know?

▲ ▲ ▲

The Peace Corps is a very good introduction to global work. There's the language training, the cultural immersion, the stress on sustainability and on working with the available resources. Really, the time I spent there was perfect for me. It was when everything came together, and I knew what I wanted to do. It might seem strange. There I was in the middle of the Liberian hinterlands. I was immersed in sad experiences. People would speak of the rainy season each year as "the hungry season." A baby living in the hut across the way from mine died, barely three months old. But it made me decide to go into development.

After two years I took off for Thailand. My future wife (who I met in Liberia) was working in rural youth development there. That was an interesting experience, trying to get work in Thailand. The Thais restricted my work permits, because even though I am an American citizen, I am of course Vietnamese-born. At that time, the Thai government only hired Thais to work inside the refugee camps. They wouldn't let me work! I finally had to come back to the US.

▲ ▲ ▲

I spent a couple years struggling to decide what to do next. I worked for a while in a medical research lab, since I have an undergraduate degree in chemistry. But the desire to do international work was still strong.

Then I learned of an opportunity to work in Vietnam, with a collaborative group of PVOs. I jumped at the chance. The first cases of AIDS were finally being acknowledged by the Vietnamese government. Through Save the Children Fund of the United Kingdom and PACT, another NGO, I had the chance to work with the government health agencies on different levels to help them deal with it. I did an evaluation for the HIV control program of SCF and its partnering organizations in the local government, to see if their peer education program worked well.

Because I knew I needed more training to get to the next level, I came back home once more to get an MPH, but I returned each summer to Ho Chi Minh City. The second summer I worked with a national AIDS committee, doing a survey of 15 provinces, looking at their capacity to work on AIDS prevention. This was also with Save the Children, a very credible and well organized agency. My last trip was in 1996, for three months. I did some exploratory work for a small PVO in Minnesota, checking out potential partners. So there was kind of an evolution for me in the sort of work I was doing, from direct service and health education, to policy analysis and program planning.

Now I work for the Minnesota Advocates for Human Rights, a small non-profit, on a project to link human rights and preventable child mortality in several countries. It's not far removed from health at all. To get to promoting health, you have to start with democracy and protection of basic human rights. I've even seen a connection between global health and voting rights, when I went to Liberia in 1997 to monitor elections.

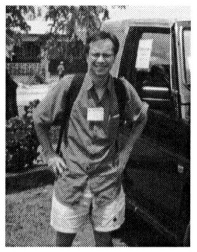

What's next for me? I'm not sure. I recently married (the same woman I met in Liberia), and we are expecting our first child next year. I'm wondering if I want to make the switch to more local work,

Huy monitored child survival, human rights and elections in East Africa.

maybe the state health department. I won't be travelling as much for a while. When you have a family you worry more about your safety. A close friend of mine was murdered overseas last year, so I have seen the terrible side of international work. But I've also seen the joy of it.

I know that whatever I do will have an international component. That's important because of who I am, my core values, my training and my professional development so far. There's a sense of restlessness that comes from having been "over there." You just feel you need to go back and share what you have, to look for your niche and do what you can.

Editor's note: Shortly after this interview, Huy was hired by the American Refugee Committe, where he is now director of global operations. He and his wife now have two children, and he says he still finds global health work challenging and rewarding.

CHAPTER EIGHT

Coming Home

Don't wait until you're overseas to read this chapter!
It's never too early to start thinking about and preparing
for your return home.

It's been an incredible experience but now it's nearing the
end. What will it be like when you get home—back to cu-
rious family and friends? Do you have to rush to find a job
and housing? Or are you going to be facing piles of paper at
work and makeup childcare responsibilities at home?

Whether you've been away for a couple of weeks or a couple
of decades, return to life in the States can be a shock to
your system and to your sensibilities. The familiar seems
strange, both to you and to those with whom you reconnect. Although they are glad to see you again, friends often
don't quite recognize you. What better proof that this work
changes you?

Even well-traveled professionals find getting back into the

swing of things a challenge. Don't underestimate the importance of preparing for the adjustment. Several groups, such as the Peace Corps, have re-entry programs to help people make the transition. If the organization that sent you overseas doesn't formally help with re-adjustment, there is much you can do on your own.

In this chapter, we'll give you pointers on how you can prepare for your return to the States, and how to build on your experience once you're back.

Before you return

Here are some pointers to start thinking about as soon as you arrive overseas—or even earlier. These will help you make the most of your personal experiences overseas.

1. Record your experiences.

The things you'll be doing while living and working overseas are far more varied than you realize now or will remember later. During your time abroad you may assume that what you're experiencing is unforgettable. It is, but trying to recall these details years later is often tough.

The more you can record about your experiences the better, from the mundane to the life-changing. Record the successes as well as the failures. This information can have many uses, both sentimental and practical. You'll refer to it when you're updating your resume, doing your final report, preparing presentations for when you get back to the States, and, of course, telling stories to your grandchildren.

There are a variety of ways to record your experiences. Keeping a daily journal or log, saving copies of your "to do" lists, or even having a small tape recorder to regularly record your thoughts and experiences are the more obvious ones. Photographs remain another good way to record your experience. Again, make a point of taking photos early on while your environment still seems new and exotic.

Be polite: ask for permission before you shoot pictures of people or places. You may find you need to pay for a picture or two. Don't take pictures of soldiers, military installations, bridges or airports. In most countries, this is against the law, and can lead to the loss of your film, camera or even your freedom.

2. Keep up connections with home.

This remains the surest cure for homesickness and can also help you reconnect when you get back. Even with the ease of the internet, you still have to write to receive. Ask your correspondents to save your letters or e-mail messages for when you return.

3. Prepare your new friends and neighbors for your departure.

In many cultures, leaving is a big deal. Follow the local traditions and take the time necessary to smooth the transition for yourselves and the people you've been working and living with. Start preparing people for your departure as soon as you know when it's going to be. The sooner the better.

Be very careful about the promises you make. In some cultures saying, "I'll see you later" means "I *will* see you later." It's a promise. So be careful when you make the commitment. Also, recognize that many people are interested in coming to live or study in the US and are looking for ways to do so. Don't get their hopes up if you can't deliver.

Be careful about offering to be a courier. People might ask you to carry mail or other things to their family and friends in the US. Establishing a set rule (i.e. whatever can fit in a shirt pocket) can help to avoid hurt feelings or miscommunication later. And watch what you do bring back. Make sure any envelopes you're given are unsealed, so you (and customs officials) can check the contents.

4. Prepare local work colleagues for your departure.

Your local counterparts should be prepared to accept your departure as a natural part of the project's evolution. Although they may be sorry to see you go, the impact of your departure can go beyond their feelings toward you, and frame their relationships with future development workers. Be sure to address their concerns about the project. What's going to happen at the project when you leave? Are you training in a replacement? Is your position going to end or is it being turned over to a local coworker? These are all questions that you need to consider well before your scheduled departure.

> **BEFORE YOUR RETURN**
> 1. Record your experiences.
> 2. Keep up connections with home.
> 3. Prepare your new friends and neighbors for your departure.
> 4. Prepare local work colleagues for your departure.
> 5. Plan for the special needs of children.
> 6. Don't get stuck at the airport.
> 7. Get your stuff home.
> 9. Use your trip home to begin your adjustment.
> 10. Take stock.

When departure day arrives, don't be surprised if there is a rather large ceremony. Be prepared to give a speech. Make a point of saying good-bye to absolutely everyone.

5. Plan for the special needs of children.

For kids who have lived a significant part of their lives overseas, the return to the US can be even more of a challenge. Language, school, TV, American culture; all can present adjustment problems to kids who may want, above all, not to seem different. Be prepared for some struggles, especially with junior-high and high-school aged children. The book *Hidden Immigrants*, by Linda Bell, (Cross-Cultural Publications) makes for fascinating reading if you wonder how a childhood overseas shapes a personality.

6. Don't get stuck at the airport.

Make sure you know what the government and the airline require for departure well before you leave for the airport. This can include exit visas, airport departure taxes in local or US currency, currency declaration forms, and restrictions on what you can take out of the country, such as antiques, religious objects, and currency. Different governments have different requirements and they can change without warning. It's also a good idea to talk with the local US Embassy if you have any questions on what you can bring in to the US, such as newly acquired pets, foods, etc.

7. Be creative with gifts for those back home.

Gifts for friends and family can set you back, unless you realize that stuff from the local market can be as colorful and exotic as crafts. Food packaging, paper goods, even household items like baskets and tableware make great gifts.

8. Think ahead about how to get your stuff home.

By nature, we humans tend to be gatherers, usually departing with far more than we brought. Before your departure, check with your airline about the size and weight limits for what you can take on board and check in. For bigger things or if you decide to take time getting home, many people ship. Check into the customs implications, the costs, and time frame for delivery.

9. Use your trip home to begin your adjustment.

Unless you're on a quick, bookended assignment and need to get back rapidly, plan to take your time getting home. Even if it's only a couple of days layover in a nice big city or a week in the country, a transitional stop can ease the lurch back into US culture.

10. Take stock.

It's easy to lose track of why we do what we do, especially when the daily grind overshadows our long-term goals. Take a look at your original motivations for global health work. Have they changed? You've just gone through a life-changing experience, so it's hard to imagine they wouldn't change in some way. Take stock, too, of the project or assignment itself. Did you accomplish what you wanted? Is the project in good hands?

Consider keeping a journal the first few weeks or months of your return. Reassessing what originally motivated you to go is step one toward closure.

The next job

While many people have jobs waiting for them when they get back home, you may be one of those who will have to wade back

> **FINDING THE NEXT JOB**
> *1. Alert the folks back home.*
> *2. Mine your overseas experience.*
> *3. Tell a good story.*
> *4. Research, research, research.*
> *5. Contact potential employers.*
> *6. Get letters from local colleagues.*

into the job market. There's a lot you can do to ease the transition to future employment, even before you depart from home.

1. Alert friends and co-workers back home that you're on the way.

Ask pals to save the employment sections of the paper for a week before your return. Some might be willing to scan the classifieds, do online searches or even set up appointments for you.

2. Mine your overseas experience.

What have you learned that will make you more employable, Stateside? The possibilities are limitless, but could include: cross-cultural communication, supervision, language fluency, community organizing, curriculum development, flexibility and program planning. Update your resume accordingly.

3. Tell a good story.

As always, a good story that relates to a job qualification can make your application stand out, especially to an employer who hasn't left the country recently.

4. Research, research, research.

If you have access to the internet, you can get newspapers and other websites listing job openings, housing and other useful information about your next home.

5. Contact potential employers.

Getting a letter or even an e-mail from overseas is still a thrill for many in the US. This can make your name memorable. Tell them when you plan to be back home, and if you can, set up a meeting.

6. Get letters of support from local counterparts.

This is a great way to demonstrate your ability and commitment to work in a cross-cultural setting.

Coming home

What a trip! You're back and it's over. Life will be different now. You've been through an experience that has physical, mental, and for some, spiritual dimensions. Take the time to rest and process your experience, if you can.

1. Stay connected with your peers overseas.

This can be one of the most important things you do in global health, especially if you can become an on-going source of support, information, opportunity for those who hosted you. E-mail access is expanding through the developing world and snail mail will go where the internet can't. The technology is there if you commit to the time.

2. Get a full medical checkup with the right doctor.

Few US doctors have seen an active case of malaria, dengue fever, or many of the parasites that might have hitched a ride home with you. You might even be hosting some of these ailments and not realize it, since many do not have immediate symptoms. You're well advised to get a full checkup soon after your return at a travel or international medicine clinic.

3. Reconnect with the home office.

Most organizations that send people overseas to work or volunteer will have some kind of a de-briefing at the end of your term. If yours doesn't, do it anyway. After you return to the States, give the home office a call and a report. The more the home office learns of the project, the better.

It's a good idea to stay connected with the organization's home office, even if there is no chance that you would go overseas with them again. Remember, the world of global health is a small one and you never know when or where old acquaintances might turn up. Home office-field program office relationships can be politically dicey. Make sure you know what you're doing if you decide to grind your ax about the project or the staff.

COMING HOME

1. *Stay connected with your peers overseas.*
2. *Get a full medical checkup with the right doctor.*
3. *Reconnect with the home office.*
4. *Prepare for "The Blank Stare."*
5. *Speak out for global health.*
6. *Practice global health at home.*
7. *Begin planning for your next trip.*

4. Prepare for "The Blank Stare."

One of the most commonly noted phenomena experienced by returnees is The Blank Stare. This is the look you get when you explain your absence, one which resembles the glassy expressions of the Pod People from Invasion of the Body Snatchers. "So what have you been up to, Sam?" "Working in a refugee camp in East Africa, Chuck." "That's nice, Sam." Click. All lights out. Conversation over.

Most Americans remain a fairly isolated lot—comfortable watching TV, going to the mall, and living life within the boundaries. What do you do when your simple response to an idle question zaps the conversation? Punt, drift into small talk, act out a flashback from that police riot in Jakarta you walked into?

Actually, a little preparation here can also help. It's a good idea to have a two minute spiel that you can use to explain your experience. Keep it simple: where you worked, what you were doing, who you were working with, what the experience was like. Don't be surprised if the conversation ends there, but expect that people do want to know something about what you've been up to. If they pursue it, you can, too. If the conversation ends, you can go back to talking about last night's game.

5. Speak out for global health and the people you served.

Not everyone looks blank when you tell them you've just returned from ten years of work in Nepal. In fact, many groups are looking for people with a story to tell. Schools (from preschools to universities), public access radio shows, churches, culture clubs and fraternal organizations (Rotary, Shriners, etc.) are just a few. Preparing and giving a presentation on your experience is one good way to build on your work.

You can also support the organization that sent you overseas by offering to speak for them when the need arises. Your experiences can enliven a pitch coming out of the fundraising department.

6. Practice global health at home.

Reread Chapter Four. There, we included a list of ways to get a taste of global health while working in your community. Many of these options can be just as useful and rewarding after your time overseas, as they were before you left. In addition, try to apply the lessons you learned overseas to your work at home. Did you learn about new models of community participation, or simpler ways to collect data? See what works in your own job.

7. *Begin planning for your next trip.*

Granted, you might not feel like it yet. But once you've lived and worked overseas, it's difficult not to think about going back. In other words, you are now an experienced global health professional, which means the longer you stay in one place, the stronger the urge to take off and help those in need becomes. So, good luck!

CAROL HALVERSON BERG
"You become a different person"

My father was a Lutheran missionary, who took his family to live in Madagascar. After their first term of seven years (before I was born), he was asked to work as Secretary for Interpretation for the American Lutheran Church headquarters in Minneapolis. All this had an effect on me: as a five year old I apparently paraded around the neighborhood saying that when I grew up I was going to be a missionary too. I already had a sense of that calling. But then I grew up very self-centered, not having a sense of any life outside of Minnesota.

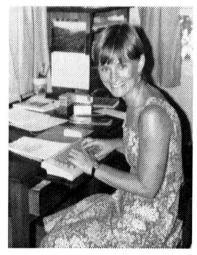

Shortly after I began nursing school, my sister died of lung cancer. I was 19. It was a tremendous shock, not only because she was young (28), a non-smoker, with a two year old son, but also because we were just beginning to be close as adults. She was my only sister. It made me re-examine my faith, values and focus in life. I could have easily become bitter from that loss but instead I felt God empowering me to recommit myself to serving my Creator and others.

Carol served as a nurse, trainer and medical missionary for ten years in Madagascar.

▲ ▲ ▲

In the spring of my final year at Lutheran Deaconess Hospital School of Nursing, a teacher told me that there was an opening for a nurse in Madagascar. I knew instantly that this is what I was supposed to do. I applied to the Lutheran church, went through the required psychological tests, was interviewed, and received a call. I was given a week-long cultural orientation to help prepare me for my new role.
I arrived in Madagascar in November 1977, and studied Malagasy for three months before starting to work in the 60-bed hospital. I was there

for three years, working as a hospital staff nurse and part-time teacher at the nursing school. The hospital was based in a very small village in the southeast tip of the island. My house was just a walk across a yard from the hospital.

When you live in a village, everybody knows you, and knows what you are doing. Kids touch your hair and skin because you are a novelty. Malagasy don't have a need for privacy like Americans. They felt so sad for me since I lived alone for many months at a time (when there were no guests or short-term volunteers staying with me). They offered to have some of their children live with me to keep me company! I loved that sense of community but I also needed time alone. I appreciated getting away every once in awhile to a small retreat cabin the church provided, about 15 miles away on the coast.

I had no security concerns then, but things have changed. A Peace Corps Volunteer was murdered in a remote village in Madagascar a few years ago. Overall, I think if you have a determined air about you and are aware of your surroundings you can be pretty safe. Generally, I stayed very healthy but I did have hepatitis A, malaria, and came home with several types of parasites (I was asymptomatic).

▲ ▲ ▲

At the time, the concept of primary health care was just taking hold, and there was no one there with advanced education in community-based health care. I realized that I needed that training, so I returned to the U.S. for a bachelor's degree in nursing, and then went to the London School of Hygiene and Tropical Medicine to get a Master of Science in Community Health. I also studied French in France for six months.

I returned to Madagascar then, to take on a new role in directing the Malagasy Lutheran Church's nursing education program. I taught in both Malagasy and French. I helped to update the curriculum to include a significant component on primary health care and on how to train village health workers. The church supports a regionally-based primary health care program which works with village health workers to do basic child growth monitoring, immunization, and teach about health topics such as the prevention and treatment of common diseases, nutrition, hygiene and sanitation, and other maternal and child health needs.

When I went back I knew it would be for a finite period. I intentionally selected a Malagasy physician and nurse to train and work with so that they could operate the nursing school on their own. There was a lot of resistance to this because expatriates are seen as more competent and reliable. After training my replacements, they asked me to stay as a co-teacher with them but I knew I needed to leave in order for others to see that they were truly in charge and doing their work competently. They continue to provide excellent leadership for the nursing school.

▲ ▲ ▲

When I came home in 1988, the needs here seemed so superficial compared to the needs overseas. It took me six months to become reoriented here and see the contributions I could make. My international experience was seen as an asset when I was hired by the Minneapolis Health Department. This is not always the case when looking for work in the US after having been overseas. Part of my job involved supervising interpreters for immigrant and refugee clients in the maternal and child health clinics. I then served as State Refugee Health Coordinator for six years with the Minnesota Department of Health. I am now Community and Public Health Manager for UCare Minnesota, a health maintenance organization.

I returned to Madagascar after I got married for a one-month trip in 1994 with my husband, David. We had been asked to do several inservices—David did some on chemical dependency treatment and prevention, and I did some on infection control and sterile technique. It was a thrill to see my Malagasy colleagues and previous nursing students doing so well, despite the struggle with increasing poverty on the island. David and I often talk about working overseas someday—whether by getting administrative leave from our jobs or retiring early.

▲ ▲ ▲

When you go overseas, you can't just step off the plane right away and get to work. You need to be intentional at first about just listening and learning from people. You can't really speed that up, even if you are only there for a short time. Before you do any good, you have to have that learning phase. So many expatriates want to get right into action. But your physical presence sometimes is just enough to encourage people, the fact that you care enough to hear about how things are going and learn from them first.

I wish there was more transfer of what we learn overseas to what we do here. Many approaches from international health work could be applied here in the US. Not just the idea of community-based care and village health workers, but also the importance of a broad-based team approach for community preventive medicine and health promotion, which requires meaningful community involvement and commitment to long-term relationships. It is truly a multi-disciplinary approach.

▲ ▲ ▲

Through intense immersion you become a different person. I've had people say that they can tell I have lived in another culture. I'm not sure why—something about the way I listen to people and respect their contributions. In learning another language, you develop an ability to listen to and understand strong accents, which helped in my work with new immigrants and interpreters. You also develop an ability to see things from other people's perspectives and world view. These skills help me a lot, every day.

Editor's note: Carol continues in her work at UCare Minnesota, where she participates in a number of initiatives aimed at reducing health disparities and is active with Global Health Ministries, a development organization run by the Lutheran Church.

Resources online

Following is a list of electronic resources on training or employment in global health. Please note that internet sites and listings change frequently.

Academic programs

www.asph.org
A listing of US-based international health academic programs, complied by the Association of Schools of Public Health.

www.healthtraining.org
A list of post-graduate training programs in global health, maintained by Medicus Mundi Switzerland, Swiss Network of Organisations for International Cooperation in Health Care.

Job, internship and volunteer listings

www.internationaljobs.org
the International Jobs Center

www.interaction.org
InterAction

www.globalhealth.org
The Global Health Council

www.reliefweb.int/vacancies
Relief Web

http://jobsearch.usajobs.opm.gov
US Government jobs

www.onlinevolunteering.org
United Nations online volunteers

www.jobs.un.org
UN agency job vacancy lists

www.who.int/employment/internship
World Health Organization internships

More on working in global health

www.ccih.org
Christian connections for International Health

www.idealist.org
Idealist.org

www.amsa.org/global
American Medical Students Association Global Action Committee

www.peacecorps.gov
US Peace Corps

www.unv.org
United Nations Volunteers

www.apha-ih.org
American Public Health Association, International Section

Useful Acronyms

AAA	American Automobile Association
AIDS	Acquired Immunodeficiency Syndrome
APHA	American Public Health Association
CARE	Cooperative for Assistance and Relief Everywhere
CDC	Centers for Disease Control and Prevention
CRS	Catholic Relief Services
FAO	Food and Agricultural Organization
ICRC	International Committee of the Red Cross
IRS	Internal Revenue Service
JSI	John Snow, Incorporated
LWR	Lutheran World Relief
MAA	Mutual Assistance Association
MPH	Master in Public Health
MSH	Management Sciences for Health
NCIH	National Council for International Health
NGO	Non-Governmental Organization
ORT	Oral Rehydration Therapy
PCV	Peace Corps Volunteer
PHC	Primary Health Care
PVO	Private Voluntary Organization
SCF	Save the Children Foundation
UN	United Nations
UNHCR	United Nations High Commissioner on Refugees
UNICEF	United Nations Children's Fund
UNV	United Nations Volunteers
USSR	Union of Soviet Socialist Republics
WHO	World Health Organization
WIC	Women, Infants and Children

What to Pack

We're not saying that you should bring all of this! In fact, one of the better reasons for going overseas is to escape most of the things on this list. Further, we recognize that needs vary from person to person, and situation to situation.

That said, here's a list of all the things you might want to bring along. Adapt it to suit your needs. It's a good idea to run your final list by someone who has either recently been where you're headed, or is currently there. They can fill you in on local availability of the key items on your packing list.

Books

dictionary/thesaurus
foreign language
    dictionary
guide books
journal or travel diary
pens and pencils (refills)
phrase book
text and reference books
writing pads

Computer stuff

computer files with your
    resume and personal
    documents
extra batteries
lap top computer
manuals and contact
    information
portable printer with
    extra ribbons/toner
voltage converter,
adapter, surge
protector

Cooking

bottle and can opener
cook book
camping food
camping stove
cooking knife
electric coil water heater
herbs and spices
plastic utensils
plastic bags

Documents

additional prescriptions
birth certificate (copy)
cash: local and US
copies of degrees and
    professional licenses
frequent flyer card
hostel card
insurance claim forms
insurance ID cards
vaccination card
international driver's
    license
inventory of your stuff
letter from physician
    describing any chronic
    conditions
letters of entry
list of credit card
    accounts
passport
personal checks
phone calling cards
photos (passport size)
plane tickets
proof of citizenship or
    green card
proof of medivac
    insurance

traveler's checks
U.S. drivers license

Electronics
batteries
battery recharger
calculator
camera (still and video)
electrical converter and
  adapters
film
tape/cd player with
  headphone
watch

First Aid
acetaminophen
antacids
antibiotics
antidiarrheal medicine
antifungal powder/cream
antihistamine
antiseptic soap
aspirin
bandages
birth control supplies
blood pressure kit
cough syrup
decongestant
hemorrhoid cream
hydrocortisone cream
ibuprofen
medical alert bracelet
oil of clove (for
  toothache)
prescription medicines
sleeping pills
thermometer
throat lozenges
tranquilizers
yeast infection medicine

Health stuff
alcohol pads or wipes

condoms
cotton swabs
dental floss
dentures and supplies
extra pair of contact
  lenses and solution
extra pair of glasses with
  prescriptions
extra tooth brushes
eye drops
hearing aid and extra
  batteries
insect repellent
iodine pills
mosquito netting
Q-tips
sanitary napkins or
  tampons
toilet tissue
tooth paste
tooth picks
tweezers
vitamins

Leisure
binoculars
blank tapes
cassettes and CDs
instruments and sheet
  music
pictures of family/friends
playing cards
telescope
walkman, CD player or
  MP3 player

Toiletries
cologne or perfume
comb and brush
cufflinks
curling iron and curlers
deodorant
hairdryer
hair remover
hair spray or gel

hangers
iron
lint remover
lotion - suntan, facial and
  body
makeup
nail polish
polish remover
razor and blades
shampoo and
  conditioner
shaving cream/powder
shoe polish and brush
soap for bathing and
  laundry
sunscreen
stain remover
towels
washcloths

Useful stuff
address book
alarm clock
battery powered short-
  wave radio
compass
duct tape
envelopes
extra set of luggage keys
flashlight
fold up luggage (extra)
luggage carts
magnifying glasses
maps
multi-use knife
plastic bags
scissors
sleeping bag or sleep sack
small metal mirror
tape measure
US postage stamps
whistle
zip lock baggies

Declaration of Alma-Ata

The International Conference on Primary Health Care, meeting in Alma-Ata this twelfth day of September in the year Nineteen hundred and seventy-eight, expressing the need for urgent action by all governments, all health and development workers and the world community to protect and promote the health of all the people of the world, hereby makes the following Declaration:

I.

The conference strongly reaffirms that health, which is a state of complete physical, mental and social wellbeing and not merely the absence of disease or infirmity, is a fundamental human right and that the attainment of the highest possible level of health is a most important worldwide social goal whose realization requires the action of many other social and economic sectors in addition to the health sector.

II

The existing gross inequiality in the health status of the people particularly between developed and developing countries as well as within countries is politically, socially and economically unacceptable and is therefore of common concern to all countries.

III.

Economic and social development, based on a New International Economic Order, is of basic importance to the fullest attainment of health for all and to the reduction of the gap between the health status of developing and developed countries. The promotion and protection of the health of the people is essential to sustained economic and social development and contributes to a better quality of life and to world peace.

IV

The people have the right and duty to participate individually and collectively in the planning and implementation of their health care.

V

Governments have a responsibility for the health of their people which can be fulfilled only by the provision of adequate health and social measures. A main social target of governments, international organizations and the whole community in the coming decades should be the attainment by all peoples of the world by the year 2000 of a level of health that will permit them to lead a socially and economically productive life. Primary health care is the key to attaining this target as part of development in the spirit of social justice.

VI

Primary health care is essential health care based on practical, scientifically sound and socially acceptable methods and technology made universally accessible to individuals and families in the community through their full participation and at a cost that the community and country can afford to maintain at every stage of their development in the spirit of self-reliance and self-determination. It forms an integral part both of the country's health system, of which it is the central function and main focus, and of the overall social and economic development of the community. It is the first level of contact of individuals, the family and community with the national health system bringing health care as close as possible to where people live and work, and constitutes the first element of a continuing health care process.

VII

Primary health care:

1. reflects and evolves from the economic conditions and the sociocultural and political characteristics of the country and its communities and is based on the application of the relevant results of social, biomedical and health services research and public health experience;

2. addresses the main health problems in the community providing promotive, preventive curative and rehabilitative services accordingly;

3. includes at least: education concerning prevailing health problems and the methods of preventing and controlling them; promotion of

food supply and proper nutrition; an adequate supply of safe water and basic sanitation; maternal and child health care, including family planning; immunization against the major infectious diseases; appropriate treatment of common diseases and injuries; and provision of essential drugs;

4. involves, in addition to the health sector, all related sectors and aspects of national and community development, in particular agriculture, animal husbandry, food, industry, education, housing, public works, communication and other sectors; and demands the coordinated efforts of all those sectors;

5. requires and promotes maximum community and individual self-reliance and participation in the planning, organization, operation and control of primary health care, making fullest use of local, national and other available resources; and to this end develops through appropriate education the ability of communities to participate;

6. should be sustained by integrated, functional and mutually-supportive referral systems, leading to the progressive improvement of comprehensive health care for all, and giving priority to those most in need;

7. relies, at local and referral levels, on health workers, including physicians, nurses, midwives, auxiliaries and community workers as applicable, as well as traditional practitioners as needed, suitably trained socially and technically to work as a health team and to respond to the expressed health needs of the community.

VIII

All governments should formulate national policies, strategies and plans of action to launch and sustain primary health care as part of a comprehensive national health system and in coordination with other sectors. To this end, it will be necessary to exercise political will, to mobilize the country's resources and to use available external resources rationally.

IX

All countries should cooperate in a spirit of partnership and service to ensure primary health care for all people since the attainment of health by people in any country directly concerns and benefits every other country. In this context the joint WHO/UNICEF report on primary health care constitutes a solid basis for the further development and operation of primary health care throughout the world.

X

An acceptable level of health for all the people of the world by the year 2000 can be attained through a fuller and better use of the world's resources, a considerable part of which is now spent on armaments and military conflicts. A genuine policy of independence, peace, detente and disarmament could and should release additional resources that could well be devoted to peaceful aims and in particular to the acceleration of social and economic development of which primary health care, as an essential part, should be allotted its proper share.

The International Conference on Primary Health Care calls for urgent and effective national and international action to develop and implement primary health care throughout the world and particularly in developing countries in a spirit of technical cooperation and in keeping with a New World Economic Order. It urges governments, WHO and UNICEF and other international organization, as well as multilateral and bilateral agencies, non-governmental organizations, funding agencies, all health workers and the whole world community to support national and international commitment to primary health care and to channel increased technical and financial support to it, particularly in developing countries. The Conference calls on the aforementioned to collaborate in introducing developing and maintaining primary health care in accordance with the spirit and content of this Declaration.